実用薬学英語

音声データダウンロードサービス付

日本薬学会編

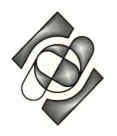

東京化学同人

まえがき

　本書は新制度の6年制薬学部で学ぶ2,3年生のための英語の教科書です．修業年限6年の薬学教育プログラムの実施に合わせて平成23年に"薬学英語入門（日本薬学会編 プライマリー薬学シリーズ1）"を刊行しましたが，本書はそれに続くものとして企画しました．6年制薬学教育を実施する各大学がカリキュラムを作成するにあたり参考とする"薬学教育モデル・コアカリキュラム"は，薬学部に対する各方面の社会的要請を考慮して再検討され，平成25年に改訂版薬学教育モデル・コアカリキュラムとして，"薬学系人材養成の在り方に関する検討会"から示されたものです．本書はコアカリキュラム改訂の理念と基本方針を理解し反映することを心掛けて作成しました．

　改訂版モデル・コアカリキュラムは薬剤師として求められる資質を明確にし，その資質を身につけるために学ぶという形をとっています．薬剤師として求められる基本的な資質として，① 薬剤師としての心構え，② 患者・生活者本来の視点，③ コミュニケーション能力，④ チーム医療への参画，⑤ 基礎的な科学力，⑥ 薬物療法における実践的能力，⑦ 地域の保健・医療における実践的能力，⑧ 研究能力，⑨ 自己研鑽，⑩ 教育能力，以上10項目があげられています．そしてこれらの資質を身につけるための目標を設定するにあたり，七つの大項目が示されました．A 基本事項，B 薬学と社会，C 薬学基礎，D 衛生薬学，E 医療薬学，F 薬学臨床，G 薬学研究 です．改訂のポイントの一つとして，薬剤師の使命，倫理観，他との信頼関係の構築を含む"A 基本事項"と，人と社会，社会保障制度，医療経済を含む"B 薬学と社会"を6年間継続して学修することがあげられています．また"F 薬学臨床"は将来の薬剤師業務の進歩を想定し，他の大項目の教育においても常に関連付けて考慮されるべきものとされています．

　このように薬剤師としての倫理観，社会性，科学を基盤として医療に貢献できる臨床の力が強く求められていることを本書に反映させるため，モデル・コアカリキュラムの大項目に続く一般目標から偏りなくテーマを選び各章の英文素材としました．

"A 基本事項"から　　　第1章：コミュニケーション
　　　　　　　　　　　第2章：生命・医療の倫理，FIP/WHO の薬学ガイドライン等
"B 薬学と社会"から　　第3章：人と社会に関わる薬剤師
"C 薬学基礎"から　　　第4章：生体分子・医薬品の化学による理解
　　　　　　　　　　　第5章：生命現象の基礎
　　　　　　　　　　　第6章：生体防御と微生物
"D 衛生薬学"から　　　第7章：健　康
　　　　　　　　　　　第8章：環　境
"E 医療薬学"と"F 薬学臨床"から
　　　　　　　　　　　第9章：神経系の疾患と薬
　　　　　　　　　　　第10章：免疫・炎症・アレルギーおよび骨・関節の疾患と薬

　　　　　　　　　　第11章：循環器系・血液系・造血系の疾患と薬
　　　　　　　　　　第12章：消化器系の疾患と薬
　　　　　　　　　　第13章：代謝系・内分泌系の疾患と薬
　　　　　　　　　　第14章：感覚器・皮膚の疾患と薬
　　　　　　　　　　第15章：病原微生物（感染症）・悪性新生物（がん）と薬
"G 薬学研究"から　　第16章：研究倫理

　本書は英語の教科書ですが，上記のように薬学の専門的内容を含んでいます．そのため第 4, 5, 9, 11, 13, 15 章は薬学専門の先生方および実際の病院薬剤師の方にご担当いただきました．その他の章についても日本薬学会の多くの先生方に専門家の視点からアドバイスをいただきました．日本薬学会の先生方にはコラム記事もご担当いただき，薬学や医学の先端的研究や技術，薬学の国際性，薬剤師の役割と倫理観などについて興味深い専門的な情報をお寄せいただきました．また米国，カナダ，ドイツ，韓国，台湾，日本の薬学部の先生方からいただいたメッセージ，およびインタビューからは，薬学的知識と臨床的能力をともに高め，広い視野をもって社会の福祉と医療に貢献することの価値と意義が伝わってきます．さらに学生の皆さんと年齢の近い，日本の薬学部を卒業し海外で活躍する薬剤師の方々はメッセージとインタビューの中で，どのように努力して英語力をみがいたか，どのようにして臨床の場で薬剤師として治療に貢献するようになったか，薬物治療の専門家としてどのように充実感を得ているかを語っています．これらを読んで薬学と英語をともに熱心に学んでいる皆さんが，世界における薬学，医学，生命科学の進歩に目を向け，医療の専門家として国際的社会に貢献し活躍する人材になってくださることを期待しています．英語力を身につけることによって，進歩の著しい世界の薬学的知識や技能を修得し，日本の患者さんの福祉にも役立つことを理解していただきたいと思います．

　本書は日本薬学会の先生方と日本薬学英語研究会（JAPE）がディスカッションを重ねて編集作成しました．刊行に当たり，東京化学同人編集部の住田六連氏，高木千織氏，丸山潤氏から深いご理解と全面的ご支援を賜りましたことに心より感謝申し上げます．多くの方々のご厚意により，薬学部学生にとって有益な英語の教科書が完成しました．編集委員一同改めてお礼を申し上げます．
　　2015 年 1 月
　　　　　　　　　　　　　　　　　　　　　　　　　　　　"実用薬学英語"編集委員一同

　本書が平成 24 年度学術研究助成基金助成金（基盤研究 C，3 年間）による研究"6 年制薬学生のための'実用薬学英語'教材の研究開発"の成果であることを付記いたします．

編集委員

入 江 徹 美	熊本大学大学院生命科学研究部 教授，薬学博士
金 子 利 雄	日本大学薬学部 教授，文学修士，M. A.(英語学)
河 野 　 円	明治大学総合数理学部 専任教授，M. A.(第二言語習得)
Eric M. Skier	東京薬科大学薬学部 准教授　M. A.(英語教授法)
竹 内 典 子*	明治薬科大学薬学部 教授，文学修士
中 村 明 弘	昭和大学薬学部 教授，薬学博士
堀 内 正 子	昭和薬科大学薬学部 准教授，修士(英語教育)

(五十音順，＊責任者)

執 筆 者

池田 年穂	慶應義塾大学薬学部 教授, 文学修士	[16章①②]
板垣 正	日本大学薬学部 専任講師, Ph.D.	[5章①②]
井原 久美子	昭和薬科大学 非常勤講師, 修士(薬学)	[13章①②]
大塚 邦子	横浜薬科大学薬学部 准教授, 博士(医学)	[9章①②, 4, 6〜9, 14章④]
大野 尚仁	東京薬科大学薬学部 教授, 薬学博士	[6章コラム]
賀川 義之	静岡県立大学薬学部 教授, 博士(医学)	[13章コラム]
金澤 洋子	昭和薬科大学薬学部 教授, M.A.(言語学), 修士(学術)	[7章①②, 1〜16章⑤]
金子 利雄	日本大学薬学部 教授, 文学修士, M.A.(英語学)	[1章①②, 1〜16章③]
亀井 美和子	日本大学薬学部 教授, 博士(薬学)	[1, 3章コラム]
川崎 郁勇	武庫川女子大学薬学部 教授, 博士(薬学)	[4章コラム]
河野 円	明治大学総合数理学部 専任教授, M.A.(第二言語習得)	[8章①②, 1〜16章⑤]
木内 祐二	昭和大学薬学部 教授, 医学博士	[11, 12章コラム]
河野 享子	京都薬科大学学生実習支援センター 助教, 理学博士	[5章①②]
河野 武幸	摂南大学薬学部 教授, 薬学博士	[10章コラム]
小佐野 博史	帝京大学薬学部 教授, 薬学博士	[14章コラム]
小林 文	昭和大学薬学部 助教, 修士(薬学)	[1章①②]
齋藤 弘明	日本大学薬学部 助教, 修士(薬学)	[4章①②]
塩田 澄子	就実大学薬学部 教授, 博士(薬学)	[15章コラム]
Eric M. Skier	東京薬科大学薬学部 准教授, M.A.(英語教授法)	[1〜16章⑤]
須川 久美子	昭和薬科大学 非常勤講師, 修士(文学)	[10章①②]
竹内 典子	明治薬科大学薬学部 教授, 文学修士	[16章①②]
田沢 恭子	明治薬科大学 非常勤講師, 修士(人文科学)	[12章①②]
玉巻 欣子	神戸薬科大学 准教授, M.A.(応用言語学), 博士(医学)	[14章①②]
徳山 尚吾	神戸学院大学薬学部 教授, 薬学博士	[9章コラム]
富岡 佳久	東北大学大学院薬学研究科 教授, 博士(薬学)	[16章コラム]
中村 明弘	昭和大学薬学部 教授, 薬学博士	[5章コラム]
平田 收正	大阪大学大学院薬学研究科 教授, 薬学博士	[7, 8章コラム]
堀内 正子	昭和薬科大学薬学部 准教授, 修士(英語教育)	[3章①②, 1〜16章④]
安原 智久	摂南大学薬学部 准教授, 博士(薬学)	[2章コラム]
山下 純	千葉大学大学院薬学研究院 客員教授, 博士(公衆衛生学)	[11章①②]
山田 惠	北海道薬科大学薬学部 教授, 博士(文学)	[6章①②]
吉田 眞紀子	医療法人鉄蕉会 亀田総合病院地域感染症疫学・予防センター 副センター長, 博士(医学)	[15章①②]
和治元 義博	北里大学一般教育部 准教授, 文学修士	[2章①②]

(五十音順)

＊ [ ]内は担当箇所: ① Reading ② Comprehension Questions ③ Grammar ④ Vocabulary ⑤ Writing

本書の使用にあたって

　本書は現在薬学部で学ぶ学生の皆さんが，将来医療に貢献する薬剤師として職責を十分に果たすための英語力を身に付けることを目標としています．そのため本書で取上げる英文素材は，皆さんが将来薬剤師として実際に読むことになる専門的英文を医学や薬学の専門誌やウェブサイトから，原文のまま引用したものです．そのため薬学の学修の進度によっては少し難解に感じられるものもあるかもしれません．特に第 11, 13, 14 章は高度に臨床的な内容を含んでいます．しかし，これらの章では薬物療法に関する問題の立て方，情報を検索しサンプルを選び分類する方法，そして的確な判断を下すに至る筋道を学ぶことができるでしょう．本当に患者さんの役に立つ薬剤師業務を行うためには，薬学に加えていかに英語の力が必要であるかを納得させられると思います．

　本書で学ばれる方の学年や薬学専門科目の進度によっては，勉強する章や練習問題を適宜選択していただいて構いませんが，確かな英語力を高めていただくために各章の英文の読み方，練習問題のねらいなどについて以下に記述させていただきます．

　1. Reading　　英語は音声を聞きながら読んでください．〔ネイティブスピーカーによる全 Reading の音声データを無料でダウンロードできます（手順および注意事項は次ページを参照）．〕薬学の専門用語がたくさん出てきますので，傍注を参考に，また英語の辞書とともに医学薬学の辞書や事典を参照しながら読むようにしてください．構文を把握し意味がわかるようになったらもう一度音声を，今度は音読しながら聞くといいでしょう．薬学の英文で使われる専門的表現や熟語的言い回しなども習得してください．

　2. Comprehension Questions　　Reading の要点を把握し内容を正しく理解できているかを確認します．正誤問題の他に英問英答の問題もあります．学術的な場面での英語による質疑応答をシミュレーションするつもりで英文を組立ててください．

　3. Grammar　　大学までに学んできた基本的英文法を薬学の専門的英文で応用できるようにします．文法は構文を把握し意味を正しく理解するために必須です．文脈に適した言い回しをすることで円滑なコミュニケーションを実現できます．

　4. Medical Vocabulary　　医療分野の専門用語とその略語を学びます．病歴の確認，医療関係者との仕事上の意思疎通，患者さんへの病状説明などのためには，専門用語の理解は欠かせません．専門用語は無理に暗記しようとするのではなく，繰返し発音しながら意味を理解することにより慣れ親しむようにしてください．

　5. Writing Exercise　　英文の薬学情報を批評的に読み，関連した研究を行って得られた検証結果を発信するためのプレゼンテーションやディスカッションの表現を学びます．実務実習や就職に使う可能性のある内容の英語表現もリハーサルしておきます．

　学生の皆さんが本書を繰返し学ぶことによって，薬学分野での英語力を高め，世界の高度な医療の正しい実現に貢献されることを願っています．

音声データについて

音声データの内容
　ファイル形式: MP3
　録音内容: 全 Reading（Track No. 1〜16）
　録音時間: 約 90 分
　ナレーター: Eric M. Skier, Erika T. Wiseberg
　（なお，音声データと同時に，別ファイルの "Doctor Kishi's Interview at UCSF"（p.6〜8）の動画もダウンロードできます．）

音声データダウンロードの手順・注意事項

　Reading ごとにトラックに分けた MP3 形式の音声ファイルを ZIP 形式で提供いたします．下記の手順でダウンロードし，パソコンで再生してご利用ください．

［ダウンロードの手順］
　1）パソコンで東京化学同人のホームページにアクセスし，書名検索などにより，"実用薬学英語" の画面を表示させる．
　2）画面最後尾の 音声ダウンロード をクリックすると下図の画面（Windows での一例）が表示されるので，下記のユーザー名およびパスワードを入力する．（本書購入者本人以外は使用できません．）

　　　　ユーザー名: **JyA81kRs4**
　　　　パスワード: **41tfYB22qS**

［保存］を選択すると，ダウンロードが始まる．

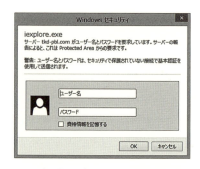

ユーザー名・パスワード入力画面の例

　※　ファイルは ZIP 形式で圧縮されていますので，解凍ソフトで解凍のうえ，ご利用ください．

［**必要な動作環境**］

　音声データのダウンロードおよび再生には，下記の動作環境が必要です．この動作環境を満たしていないパソコンでは正常にダウンロードおよび再生ができない場合がありますので，ご了承ください．

OS：Microsoft Windows Vista/7/8/8.1，Mac OS X 10.7/10.8/10.9（日本語版サービスパックなどは最新版）
推奨ブラウザ：Microsoft Internet Explorer，Safari など
コンテンツ再生：Microsoft Windows Media Player など

［**音楽 CD プレイヤーで再生するには**］

　音楽 CD プレイヤーなどで再生する場合には，パソコン上で適切なアプリケーション（Windows Media Player など）を用いて，オーディオ CD（データ CD ではない）を作成していただく必要があります．CD は 1 枚では入りきらないので 2 枚ご準備ください．オーディオ CD の作成の仕方は，各アプリケーションの説明書でご確認ください．弊社でのお客様ごとの個別対応はいたしかねますのでご了承ください．

［**データ利用上の注意**］

・本音声データのダウンロードおよび再生に起因して使用者に直接または間接的障害が生じても株式会社東京化学同人はいかなる責任も負わず，一切の賠償などは行わないものとします．
・本音声データは著作権上の保護を受けています．本音声データの一部あるいは全部について，いかなる方法においても無断で複写，複製し，有償・無償を問わず配布，配信することを禁じます．

目　　次

Chapter 1　Motivational Interviewing（MI）—Four Guiding Principles
（動機付け面接法 — 四つの基本原則）············1
　Interview　Doctor Kishi's Interview at UCSF················6
Chapter 2　Good Pharmacy Practice（薬局業務規範）············9
　Message to You　UIC での経験を通して················15
Chapter 3　Creating an Environmentally Friendly Pharmacy
（環境に配慮した薬局をつくる）············16
Chapter 4　Targeted Cancer Therapies（標的がん治療薬）············22
　Message to You　Pharmacy Practice and Education in Alberta················27
Chapter 5　Insulin（インスリン）············30
　Interview　My Path to JICA················35
Chapter 6　The Immune System（免疫系）············37
Chapter 7　Low-Fat Diet Not a Cure-All（低脂肪ダイエットは万能薬にあらず）············42
　Message to You　German Pharmacy Education················47
Chapter 8　Air Quality Deteriorating in Many of the World's Cities
（世界の多くの都市で悪化する大気環境）············49
　Interview　Working as a JICA Volunteer in Ghana················55
Chapter 9　Mental Health of Older Adults, Addressing a Growing Concern
（高齢者の精神保健，膨らむ懸念に対応するために）············57
Chapter 10　Rheumatoid Arthritis（関節リウマチ）············63
　Message to You　Pharmacy Education in Korea················68
Chapter 11　Dabigatran Versus Warfarin in Patients With Mechanical Heart Valves
（機械弁置換手術を受けた患者でのワルファリンと対比した
ダビガトラン投与試験）············70
　Message to You　Licensed to Work as a Pharmacist in Both Japan and America············76
Chapter 12　More Drugs Show Promise in Fighting Hepatitis C
（C 型肝炎との闘いに有望な薬が新たに登場）············78
Chapter 13　End of the Road: Diabetes Care When Insulin May Not Be an Option
（インスリンの使用が困難な場合の糖尿病治療 — 希望はあるのか）············84
　Message to You　Evolution of Pharmacy Education in Taiwan············89
Chapter 14　Drugs Acting on the Eye（眼に作用する薬）············91
　Message to You　A Message From a Pharmacist Specializing in Cancer
to the Future Pharmacists of Japan············96

Chapter 15 Primary Isoniazid Prophylaxis Against Tuberculosis
　　　　　　in HIV-Exposed Children （HIV に曝露された子供における
　　　　　　　　　　　　イソニアジドによる結核の一次予防）　…98

Chapter 16 On Being a Scientist: Responsible Conduct in Research
　　　　　　　　　　　　（科学者の責任ある研究活動について）………103

　Message to You　Pharmacists as Health Care Providers
　　　　　　　　　　　in the United States—Current Status………108

Chapter 1
Motivational Interviewing (MI)
Four Guiding Principles

1・1 Reading

> この章では，motivational interviewing (MI) の指針を読んでみよう．Stephen Rollnick, William R. Miller, Christopher C. Butler が紹介した MI とは，相談者が自分で変わろうとするきっかけや行動変化に対し援助を行う方法である．国内では医学，福祉，教育，心理学などの幅広い領域で活用されている．薬剤師を目指す薬学生が学ぶコミュニケーションスキルとして MI の指針を学んでみよう．

motivational interviewing (MI) 動機付け面接法

If you are a health care professional, you probably have many conversations about behavior change in the course of your typical work day. What is often less clear is how a practitioner should approach this topic.

health care professional 医療従事者
practitioner 開業医などの医療専門家

The practice of MI, or motivational interviewing, has four guiding principles: (1) to resist the righting reflex, (2) to understand and explore the patient's own motivations, (3) to listen with empathy, and (4) to empower the patient, encouraging hope and optimism. These four principles can be remembered by the acronym RULE: Resist, Understand, Listen, and Empower.

righting reflex 正したいという反射的な反応

R: Resist the righting reflex

People who enter helping professions often have a powerful desire to set things right, to heal, to prevent harm and promote well-being. When seeing someone headed down the wrong path, they will usually want to get out in front of the person and say, "Stop! Turn back! There is a better way!" This is a laudable motivation; it is often what calls people into service to others.

PRACTITIONER: Well, if you did decide to exercise more, that would not only help your knee but also help you lose weight and improve your mood, you know. Exercise makes people slimmer, fitter, and feel better.

PATIENT: Yes, I know all that. But I can't help thinking that if I exercise while my knee hurts, even with gentle things like swimming, that I am doing more damage to it, despite what you say about those studies you read.

This acting out of the patient's internal dilemma might be therapeutic in some way were it not for another well-documented basic principle of human nature. In sum, if you are arguing for change and your patient is resisting and arguing against it, you're in the wrong role. You are taking all the good lines. It is the patient who should be voicing the argument. MI is about evoking those arguments from the patient, and that means first suppressing what may seem like the right thing to do—the righting reflex.

U: Understand your patient's motivations

It is the patient's own reasons for change, and not yours, that are most likely to trigger behavior change. And so a second guiding principle is to be interested in the patient's own concerns, values, and motivations. In MI one proceeds in a way that evokes and explores patients' perceptions about their current situations and their own motivations for change. This may sound like a prolonged process, but it need not be. It can be done within the normal length of your consultation. We believe, in fact, that if your consultation time is limited, you are better off asking patients why they would want to make a change and how they might do it rather than telling them that they should. It is the patient, rather than you, who should be voicing the arguments for behavior change.

L: Listen to your patient

MI involves at least as much listening as informing. Perhaps the normal expectations of a health care consultation are that the practitioner has the answers and will give them to the patients. Often you do have answers, and patients come to you for this expertise. When it comes to behavior change, though, the answers most likely lie within the patient, and finding them requires some listening. Good listening is actually a complex clinical skill. It requires more than asking questions and keeping quiet long enough to hear patients' replies.

E: Empower your patient

It is increasingly clear that outcomes are better when patients take an active interest and role in their own health care. A fourth guiding principle in MI is empowerment—helping patients explore how they can make a difference in their own health. Patients in essence become your consultants on their own lives and on how best to accomplish behavior change. An important role for you in this process is to support their hope that such change is possible and can make a difference in their health. A patient who is active in the consultation, thinking aloud about the why and how of change, is more likely to do something about this afterward. You, the practitioner, are an expert in facilitating the patients' bringing their expertise to the consultation.

出典：S. Rollnick, W. R. Miller, C. C. Butler "Motivational Interviewing in Health Care: Helping Patients Change Behavior", 7〜10（2008）より The Guilford Press の許可を得て転載；許可は米国 Copyright Clearance Center を通して取得した．Copyright ©2008 The Guilford Press. All rights reserved.

1・2 Comprehension Questions

Match each of the following principles with its meaning below.

1. Resist the Righting Reflex   (   )
2. Understand Your Patient's Motivation (   )
3. Listen to Your Patient   (   )
4. Empower Your Patient   (   )

a. 患者が変わろうとする気持ちを傾聴すること．
b. 患者に変わりたい，変わりたくないというジレンマがあること．
c. 医療従事者は，患者が変化していく過程での支えになること．
d. 患者が変わろうとするきっかけを理解すること．
e. 患者の動機付けに興味をもつこと．

1・3 Grammar

Identify the grammatical error, if any, in each sentence and rewrite it in a correct way.

Target ➤ Nouns (singular and plural forms)

1. Though research is ongoing, the FDA says that available scientific evidences—including WHO findings released May 17, 2010—shows no increased health risk due to radiofrequency (RF) energy, a form of electromagnetic radiation that is emitted by cell phones.
2. Scientific knowledges gained through these activities also allows CDER to respond swiftly to unforeseen public health emergencies.
3. Certain data and information contained in food additive petitions are available for public disclosure, while other data is not.
4. *Salmonella* species can cause serious and sometimes fatal infections in young children, frail or elderly people, and others with weakened immune systems.
5. The excessive synthesis of multiple gene products derived from the overexpression of the genes present on chromosome 21 are thought to underlie both the dysmorphic features and the pathogenesis of the neurological, immunologic, endocrine, and biochemical abnormalities that are characteristic of DS.

CDER Center for Drug Evaluation and Research (FDA医薬品評価センター)

DS Down syndrome (ダウン症候群)

1・4 Medical Vocabulary
▶ 学会・組織の名称と略語

Match each of the following abbreviated words with its meaning below and then translate the word into Japanese.

1. CDC ( ) _____
2. FIP ( ) _____
3. WMA ( ) _____
4. WHO ( ) _____
5. FDA ( ) _____
6. NIH ( ) _____
7. PMDA ( ) _____
8. MSF ( ) _____

a. World Medical Association
b. Food and Drug Administration
c. Médicine Sans Frontières [F*]
d. Centers for Disease Control and Prevention
e. World Health Organization
f. Federation Internationale Pharmaceutique [F]
g. National Institutes of Health
h. Pharmaceutical and Medical Devices Agency

＊　フランス語

1・5　Writing Exercise
▶ **Self-Introduction of an "Entry Sheet"**

You are filling in an "entry sheet" for an intern job at a pharmaceutical company. Write a brief self-introduction.

Hints！
薬学生：student pharmacist（よりプロらしい），pharmacy student
3年生：3rd-year student

COLUMN

薬剤師による動機付け面接

　どんなに優れた薬が開発されたとしても，きちんと使用されなければ期待する効果を得ることはできません．入院患者の場合，医療従事者が治療の管理をしますが，通院患者の場合は，患者が自分自身で管理をするか，家族や介護者に援助してもらうことになります．

　糖尿病や高血圧などの生活習慣病では，自覚症状がない場合も多く，長期間の薬物療法を自己管理で正しく継続するのは大変なことです．医療従事者が患者のモチベーションを高め，治療を中断させないように関わる必要がありますが，そこで大事なことが治療薬に関する情報交換だけではない，患者との対話です．薬局で1～2カ月ごとに薬を受取りに来る患者と，薬剤師が会話できる時間はほんの数分間ですが，数分間であっても，患者をエンパワーメントし，自己管理能力を高めることができるといわれています．そのポイントが，動機付け面接法です．薬剤師が動機付け面接法を身に付けることで，通院患者の治療効果の向上が期待できます．

（亀井美和子）

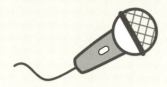
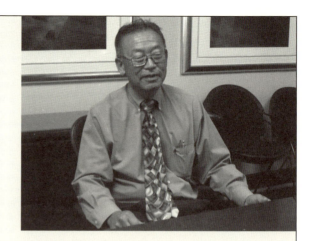

Doctor Kishi's Interview at UCSF*

Skier: Hello. May I have your name?

Kishi: I'm Don Kishi.

Skier: And what's your educational background?

Kishi: I went to, after high school, I went to University of California Davis, which is near Sacramento, and after that, two years at that school, I came to University of California San Francisco, Scholl of Pharmacy.

Skier: What did you study in UC Davis?

Kishi: General.

Skier: Oh, OK.

Kishi: General education requirements to get into pharmacy school.

Skier: So, as an undergrad at UC Davis, you already knew that you wanted to come to pharmacy school?

Kishi: I did know that I wanted to come to pharmacy school. I understood that one of my goals was to help people. I didn't want to be a surgeon. I had a friend whose father owned a pharmacy and so I talked with him and some other people. And I made a decision this is what I wanted to do.

Skier: You were eighteen years old?

Kishi: I was eighteen. I was actually before that, it was during high school that I was gathering information and made a decision to go to pharmacy school.

Skier: How about your work experience after you graduated?

Kishi: I was very lucky. When I graduated it was beginning of the new part of our profession which is clinical pharmacy. And so I was able to become involved with that as it was beginning to develop. And so we were trying new things, new roles for pharmacists, new techniques. One of the most important thing was that we were able to move from the basement of the hospital up to the floor, the nursing

---

* このインタビューの動画も，Reading の音声ファイルと同時にダウンロードできます．ダウンロードの方法についてはxページを参照してください．

unit, the ward and to interact with the physicians and the nurses and the patients in the environment of the ward and that also provided us the opportunity to not only speak with those people but also it gave us access to the medical records so that we could begin doing some activities such as monitoring of the patients and their drug therapy.

Skier: But, in particular, so you were a hospital pharmacist?

Kishi: I was a hospital pharmacist, yes.

Skier: And then, when did you become an educator?

Kishi: Well, we actually did both because as we developed the role of the pharmacist on the ward. I also and my colleagues also began to teach students on the ward and then also as we developed the therapeutics course, the clinical course, we started to give lectures within those courses about diseases and how to use drugs appropriately within those diseases.

Skier: I see. What do you think about your current work situation?

Kishi: In between being a practicing pharmacist and right now I am associate dean for students and curriculum in the school. But in between I also was a manager in the hospital pharmacy I was also a vice chairman in the department clinical pharmacy, which is in the school site. I practiced on general surgery services, general medicine services, kidney transplant services, neurology services, neurosurgery services all during that interim time period. I also let's see, I was also in neurology clinic and I was able to manage the drug therapy of patients who had epilepsy or seizures and so I had a group of patients that I was taking care of.

Skier: And that was very satisfying for you?

Kishi: Very very satisfying. You learn how to interact with patients as well as with health care colleagues. You learn how to communicate effectively. I even use more Spanish now, when I was in the clinic, because a lot of my population that I was taking care of were Spanish speakers. So I had to learn and brush up on my high school Spanish.

Skier: OK. Interesting. Would you mind say something to the students of Japan, pharmacy students.

Kishi: (To) student pharmacists in Japan? There are a few things that I would like to say. One is that communication skills and interpersonal skills are very vital to your success as a pharmacist. I am not just talking about what has happened in the United States but also in developing new roles for pharmacists in the hospital, in clinics in the community, for home care, a variety of different kinds of settings, communication skills, interacting with people becomes very important. I would say also, since many people now in the world now speak English that English skills are also very important to your practice, because you as …, even though you may be practicing in Japan, you will get many visitors from different countries many of whom speak English as their second language but you should be able to communicate with them. I think the other thing that is true for Japan is your population is getting older and so not only respecting your elders but understanding how they differ from your younger population is also important. They are different in terms of disease states. They are different in terms of metabolism of drugs so it becomes important to understand what's going on in their lives also. The last thing I would say is that the future of Japanese pharmacy is in your hands. You will make the changes. You will make the profession go forward. You have to be willing to climb many mountains and obstacles to make that may happen, but if just remember that the people you are serving are your patients, it's not the physicians, it's not the nurses, it's not just your colleagues, but it's your patients, and your patient should always be number one motivator for you to do something. OK, so please Ganbatte Kudasai!

Skier: Thank you very much!

                                            Don T. Kishi, PharmD
                                            Associate Dean
                                            Office of Student & Curricular Affairs
                                            Health Sciences Clinical Professor
                                            Department of Clinical Pharmacy in UCSF

Chapter 2

Good Pharmacy Practice

2・1 Reading

2011年，国際薬剤師・薬学連合（International Pharmaceutical Federation: FIP）および世界保健機関（World Health Organization: WHO）により，薬局業務規範（Good Pharmacy Practice: GPP）に関する FIP/WHO 共同ガイドラインが策定された．六つのセクションから成る本文には，薬局業務規範の中心的な理念，定義，要件，規範の設定などが述べられている．ここでは，第3セクション"定義"と第4セクション"要件"を読み，薬局業務規範の一端を学習しよう．将来薬剤師として働くうえできっと役に立つはずである．

 Track 2

Definition of good pharmacy practice

GPP is the practice of pharmacy that responds to the needs of the people who use the pharmacists' services to provide optimal, evidence-based care. To support this practice it is essential that there be an
5 established national framework of quality standards and guidelines.

optimal　最善の
evidence-based　エビデンス（科学的根拠）
quality standard　品質基準

Requirements of good pharmacy practice

・GPP requires that a pharmacist's first concern in all settings is the welfare of patients.

in all settings　あらゆる状況において

・GPP requires that the core of the pharmacy activity is to help patients
10 make the best use of medicines. Fundamental functions include the supply of medication and other health-care products of assured quality, the provision of appropriate information and advice to the patient, administration of medication, when required, and the monitoring of the effects of medication use.

administration of medication　医薬品の投与

15 ・GPP requires that an integral part of the pharmacist's contribution is

the promotion of rational and economic prescribing, as well as dispensing.

- GPP requires that the objective of each element of pharmacy service is relevant to the patient, is clearly defined and is effectively communicated to all those involved. Multidisciplinary collaboration among health-care professionals is the key factor for successfully improving patient safety.

In satisfying these requirements, the following conditions are necessary:

- the well-being of patients should be the main philosophy underlying practice, even though it is accepted that ethical and economic factors are also important;
- pharmacists should have input into decisions about the use of medicines. A system should exist that enables pharmacists to report and to obtain feedback about adverse events, medicine-related problems, medication errors, misuse or medicine abuse, defects in product quality or detection of counterfeit products. This reporting may include information about medicine use supplied by patients or health professionals, either directly or through pharmacists;
- the relationship with other health professionals, particularly physicians, should be established as a therapeutic collaborative partnership that involves mutual trust and confidence in all matters relating to pharmacotherapy;
- the relationship between pharmacists should be one of colleagues seeking to improve pharmacy service, rather than acting as competitors;
- in reality, organizations, group practices and pharmacy managers should accept a share of responsibility for the definition, evaluation and improvement of quality;
- the pharmacist should be aware of essential medical and

pharmaceutical information (i.e. diagnosis, laboratory test results and medical history) about each patient. Obtaining such information is made easier if the patient chooses to use only one pharmacy or if the patient's medication profile is available;

- the pharmacist needs evidence-based, unbiased, comprehensive, objective and current information about therapeutics, medicines and other health-care products in use, including potential environmental hazards caused by disposal of medicines' waste;

- pharmacists in each practice setting should accept personal responsibility for maintaining and assessing their own competence throughout their professional working lives. While self-monitoring is important, an element of assessment and monitoring by the national pharmacy professional organizations would also be relevant in ensuring that pharmacists maintain standards and comply with requirements for continuous professional development;

- educational programmes for entry into the profession should appropriately address both current and foreseeable changes in pharmacy practice; and

- national standards of GPP should be specified and should be adhered to by practitioners.

At the national or appropriate (e.g. state or provincial) level, it is necessary to establish:

- A legal framework that:
  - defines who can practice pharmacy;
  - defines the scope of pharmacy practice;
  - ensures the integrity of the supply chain and the quality of medicines.
- A workforce framework that:
  - ensures the competence of pharmacy staff through continuing

2. Good Pharmacy Practice

professional development (CPD or continuing education (CE)) programmes;

- defines the personnel resources needed to provide GPP.

・An economic framework that:

- provides sufficient resources and incentives that are effectively used to ensure the activities undertaken in GPP.

出 典：*Joint FIP/WHO Guidelines on Good Pharmacy Practice*: *Standards for quality of pharmacy services*, International Pharmaceutical Federation のウェブサイト〔http://www.fip.org/www/uploads/database_file.php?id=331&table_id=（2015年1月現在）〕より転載. WHO Technical Report Series, No.961, 2011.

2・2　Comprehension Questions

Fill in the blanks with words which begin with the given letters.

1. The relationship between pharmacists should be one of coworkers who seek to （im　　　）pharmacy service, rather than to （com　　　）with each other.
2. Pharmacists should know the （es　　　）medical and pharmaceutical information about each （pa　　　）, but accessing such information would be more （dif　　　）if the patient chooses to use two or more （phar　　　）or if the patient's （med　　　）（pro　　　）is not available.
3. Pharmacists and other health professionals must establish a （ther　　　）collaborative partnership which is necessary for them to share （mu　　　）trust and be （con　　　）in all matters relating to pharmacotherapy.
4. The key factor for successful （im　　　）of patient safety is （multi　　　）collaboration among health-care professionals.
5. Working as （pro　　　）, pharmacists in each practice setting should be personally （re　　　）for maintaining and assessing their own competence.

2・3　Grammar

Numbers 1 and 2 are stylistically fragile in terms of science writing. The rest of the sentences are grammatically or stylistically wrong. Find and fix each error.

Target ▶ Pronoun

1. It is concluded that smoking has an impact on the periodontal status and mRNA expression of MMP-8 and TIMP-1 in chronic periodontitis patients.
2. It is found that RB (Rohon-Beard) and MTN (mesencephalic trigeminal nucleus) neurons express a core set of genes indicative of sensory neurons.
3. Specialist care is needed for a small proportion of individuals with complicated depression or them who do not respond to first-line treatments.
4. The amount of buprenorphine in a dose of ZUBSOLV® is not the same as the

amount of buprenorphine in other medicines that contain buprenorphine.
5. The malaria parasite that impacts mice used in lab tests is structurally different from one infecting humans.

2・4 Medical Vocabulary
▶ 処方箋の略語 (1)

Match each of the following abbreviated words with its meaning below and then translate the word into Japanese.

1. a.c.   (   ) _____
2. Amp   (   ) _____
3. anal.   (   ) _____
4. Aq. dest. (   ) _____
5. b.i.d.   (   ) _____
6. Cap, cap (   ) _____
7. h.d.   (   ) _____
8. i.c.   (   ) _____

a. Aqua destillate [L*]　　　　　　　　　　　　　　　　　＊　ラテン語
b. inter cibos [L]
c. ampule
d. analgesia [L]
e. ante cibum (cibos) [L]
f. capsule
g. hora decubitus [L]
h. bis in die [L]

2・5 Writing Exercise
▶ **Presentation on your university**

You are to introduce your university at a student conference. Explain the history and location of your university.

> Hi everyone. Today, I will introduce my university to you.

COLUMN

薬剤師になるという意味

　薬剤師法には，"薬剤師は調剤，医薬品の供給その他薬事衛生をつかさどる"，"薬剤師でない者は，販売又は授与の目的で調剤してはならない"と明記されている．薬剤師にとって特別の意味をもつ"調剤"とは具体的には何か．薬剤師会の定めた調剤指針によれば，調剤とは"薬物療法の個別最適化と評価，フィードバック"である．患者一人一人の病状，訴え，生活の実態，価値観に合わせ，目の前の患者の人生に最も貢献する薬物療法に介入し，効果を見極め，患者と医師にその内容を伝達していくことである．これは誰にでもできることではない．したがって国は一般には"調剤"を禁止し，能力が認められ薬学部を卒業し国家試験に合格した者だけに，免許として"調剤"を行う許可を与える．薬剤師になるということは，一般には禁止された行為を特別に許された誇りと使命感を掲げて，"公衆衛生の向上及び増進に寄与し，もつて国民の健康な生活を確保する"任務を負うということである．

〈安原智久〉

UICでの経験を通して

　1997年秋から1998年夏までイリノイ大学シカゴ校（UIC）にてPharm Dコース（教養課程2年終了後の4年間の専門課程）の3年次の講義や演習と4年次の臨床研修を体験して感じたことをお話します。留学前に日本で臨床系大学院修士・博士課程において大学病院の病棟薬剤師業務を研修し、薬剤師の役割というものを理解した上でUICに向かいましたので、前半の3年次の薬物治療学、医薬品情報学などの講義や症例解析演習については、語学のハンディはあったものの日本での教育と分厚い英文（原著）のテキストに助けられました。後半の4年次の臨床研修は、一般内科から始まりました。初日から他の学生同様に担当患者が数名割り当てられましたが、語学のハンディだけでなく、患者情報を得るためのPCの使い方も知らない私は他の学生と同じようにできずショックを受けました。さらに、それまで私が日本で研修してきた病棟薬剤師の業務は、回診や病棟ミーティングで患者の治療方針を把握し薬物治療に関して提案をしたり、患者の処方を確認し医師に問い合わせをしたり、患者に服薬指導を行い効果や副作用の確認後その記録を残すというもので、けっして米国に劣らないという自負があったのですが、UICでは薬剤師が入院時サマリーおよび退院時サマリーを記入しカルテにとじていたのです。そのため、研修初日から入院したばかりの患者の情報を集めなければなりませんでした。日本だとカルテを見れば医師や看護師によって集められた情報があるのですが、UICでは入院したばかりの患者の情報はカルテを見ても参考になる情報が得らないことも多く、自分でインタビューを行い、入院時サマリーを作成する必要があったのです。入院時のサマリーには基本的に患者の入院までの経緯、OTC薬も含めた薬歴、アレルギー・副作用歴、身長・体重、腎機能、アドヒアランス、投薬の必要性、TDMが必要な患者についてはそのレベルおよび解析、薬物相互作用、モニタリングパラメーターについて問題点ごとに記入することになっていました。この記録を参考に医師が投与設計も行っていましたので業務のスピードも要求されたわけです。体当たりで研修はなんとか無事に終えることができました。

　その他の研修を通して求められる薬剤師業務は病棟やチームによって多少異なることを知りましたし、米国と日本では診療報酬の制度も異なるため、UICで体験した病棟薬剤師業務を単純に日本と比較することはできません。しかし、すべての薬剤師に共通していえることは、新薬情報や新しい治療法を検討する場合には英語の文献を利用する必要があり、情報を正しく評価するために英語能力は必須だということです。

　He/She who graduated yesterday and stops learning today, will be uneducated tomorrow. 常に学ぶということを忘れずにいたいものです。

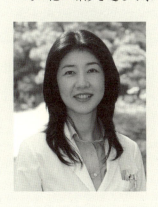

明治薬科大学 准教授
門田佳子

Chapter 3
Creating an Environmentally Friendly Pharmacy

3・1 Reading

> 1960年代，Rachel Carson は "Silent Spring（沈黙の春）" で農薬などの化学物質の危険性を訴え，環境保護運動の先駆けとなった．分析技術が進歩した1990年代以降，本来は人や動物の病気の予防と治療に欠かせない薬剤が飲料水中に見つかると，この問題はみなの注目を集めた．今，"市井の科学者" である薬剤師には新たな役割が求められている．一緒に考えてみよう．

impact 影響（力）
pharmacy practice 薬局実務
pharmaceutical 薬剤, 医薬品
personal-care products パーソナルケア製品〈化粧品, 衛生用品など〉
contaminate 汚染する
water supply 水道, 飲料水
soundness 健全性

going green 環境に配慮したあり方

Most studies relating to the impact of pharmacy practice on the environment focus on concerns regarding pharmaceuticals and personal-care products (PCPs) contaminating our water supply. In many ways, however, the business of pharmacy is much like other enterprises, and it is worthwhile to examine the environmental soundness of processes and practices. Moreover, as healthcare professionals providing both service and product components, pharmacists have unique opportunities to introduce their patients and customers to more environmentally appropriate practices in a variety of areas.

This article is intended to assist pharmacists in identifying areas in which they can consider "going green." It examines environmental issues relating to pharmacy practice, as well as the store or practice site. It also discusses the important educational role that pharmacists can play in the community. In addition, resources are provided for pharmacists to obtain more detailed information.

getting started はじめに

Getting started

Identifying and tackling environmental issues in a busy pharmacy might seem like a daunting task. However, taking one small step can make a big difference; it can motivate staff and patients/customers to integrate consideration of environmental issues into daily practice and daily life. Pharmacists could begin by identifying a single environmental issue that relates to their processes or practice, and adopt measures to address this issue.

What are pharmacists already doing?

Community health surveillance

Pharmacists are in an ideal position to identify community outbreaks due to improper environmental management. For example, two outbreaks due to contaminated water (Walkerton, Ont. and the Battlefords area of Saskatchewan) affected thousands of people in entire communities. Pharmacists assisted public health officials in identifying these outbreaks by noting the spike in the sale of antinauseants, antidiarrheals and rehydration products.

Waste diversion
Appropriate use of medication
Minimize wastage
Promote environmentally friendly manufacturing

What more can pharmacists do?

Pharmacists sell numerous medications and consumer products. The environmental risks associated with these agents, singly or in combination—including the risk to human or animal health when they enter our water supply—is not known. Accordingly, it is sound practice to remind consumers not to overuse these products, and to offer a selection of alternative, more environmentally friendly products.

3. Creating an Environmentally Friendly Pharmacy

Studies that examine the environmental impact of pharmaceuticals and PCPs typically do not consider the role of nonmedicinal ingredients in medications and consumer products. First, consider whether these agents are essential components of a product. If not, perhaps the pharmacy could stock similar products that contain fewer ingredients and that are more environmentally appropriate.

The pharmacist as environmental educator
· As part of routine patient counselling, make customers aware of the environmental consequences of their decisions to consume pharmaceuticals and personal care products.
· Advise patients to bring back any unused prescription, nonprescription or alternative medicines to the pharmacy for proper disposal.
· Include an accessory label on all prescriptions that says "bring unused portion back to pharmacy for disposal;" alternatively, include this information on patient handouts.
· Encourage patients to use OTC products at the lowest effective dosage (and to bring back outdated drugs for disposal).
· Remind patients that personal care products enter our water supply. Suggest that they use smaller volumes or use brands that have less environmental impact.
· Help customers decipher product labels.   - Many terms are used that confuse the consumer (e.g., fragrance free, unscented, hypoallergenic, not tested on animals,

preservative-free, dermatologist tested, natural vs. synthetic). What do these terms really mean? Answers can be found, for example, at Health Canada's Cosmetics: FAQ

dermatologist tested 皮膚科医によるテスト済みの

- Include environmental issues in the services you provide.
  - Discuss environmental issues specific to medications, personal care products and other chemicals.
  - When you talk to groups (e.g., patients, students, seniors) about medications, include environmental impact as part of your discussion.
  - Work with your municipality to offer free recycling opportunities for customers (e.g., hold medication return days).
  - Encourage staff and customers to bring "greening" ideas to you.
  - Make it fun; help your customers calculate their ecological footprint, (e.g., take the quiz at www.globalfootprintnetwork.org).

municipality 地方自治体, 市(町)当局

ecological footprint エコロジカルフットプリント〈環境用語. 人間活動により消費される生態系資源の量を土地面積として表す〉

- Above all, make sure your patients know that one person can indeed make a difference in protecting our environment.

出 典: J. Campbell, "Creating an environmentally friendly pharmacy", *Pharmacypractice*, *March/April 2008*, 16〜17, 19〜20 より転載. Copyright ©2009-2014 Rogers Publishing Limited. All rights reserved.

3・2 Comprehension Questions

Answer the following questions in English.

1. What is a major concern for pharmacy studies on environmental issues?

　　_____

2. Why did the author write this article?

　　_____

3. How can pharmacists in a busy pharmacy take a step to wards identifying and tackling environmental issues?

　　_____

4. What happened in Walkerton, Ontario and the Battlefords area of Saskatchewan?

_____

5. Describe an example related to each of the four subtitles, *Waste diversion*, *Appropriate use of medication*, *Minimize wastage*, and *Promote environmentally friendly manufacturing*.

_____

_____

_____

_____

3・3 Grammar

Put an appropriate article, either *a*, *an*, or *the*, in the parentheses to make each sentence meaningful.

Target ▶ Article

1. Over (   ) past four decades, the increased use of fertility treatments in the United States has been associated with a substantial rise in the rate of multiple births.
2. The viral envelope glycoprotein GP is either (   ) component of, or the sole viral antigen in many ebolavirus candidate vaccines.
3. The genus *Ebolavirus* is (   ) member of the family *Filoviridae*. *Ebolavirus* includes five species: *Zaire ebolavirus*, *Sudan ebolavirus*, *Tai Forest ebolavirus*, *Reston ebolavirus*, and *Bundibugyo ebolavirus*.
4. Removing the rabies virus at the site of the infection by chemical or physical means is (   ) effective means of protection.
5. The number of people visually impaired from infectious diseases has reduced in (   ) last 20 years according to global estimates.

3・4 Medical Vocabulary

▶ 処方箋の略語（2）

Match each of the following abbreviated words with its meaning below and then translate the word into Japanese.

1. P.O., p.o.   (   ) _____
2. Pulv.   (   ) _____
3. Supp, sup   (   ) _____
4. t.i.d.   (   ) _____
5. ss   (   ) _____

3. Creating an Environmentally Friendly Pharmacy

6. Syr, syr　　　　（　）＿＿＿＿＿＿＿＿＿＿＿＿＿＿＿＿＿＿

7. t.m.　　　　　 （　）＿＿＿＿＿＿＿＿＿＿＿＿＿＿＿＿＿＿

8. Ug., ung., ungt.（　）＿＿＿＿＿＿＿＿＿＿＿＿＿＿＿＿＿＿

a. Pulvis ［L*］　　　　　　e. syrup　　　　　　　　　＊　ラテン語
b. Unguentum ［L］　　　　f. ter in die ［L］
c. per os ［L］　　　　　　g. tota massa ［L］
d. semis ［L］　　　　　　 h. suppository

3・5 Writing
▶ **Expressing career plans**

Suppose you are at a job interview. What would you answer when asked, "What is your future goal as a pharmacist/researcher/healthcare professional?"

In the future, I hope to ＿＿＿＿＿＿＿＿＿＿＿＿＿＿＿＿＿＿＿＿＿＿

＿＿＿＿＿＿＿＿＿＿＿＿＿＿＿＿＿＿＿＿＿＿＿＿＿＿＿＿＿＿＿＿＿＿＿

＿＿＿＿＿＿＿＿＿＿＿＿＿＿＿＿＿＿＿＿＿＿＿＿＿＿＿＿＿＿＿＿＿＿＿

＿＿＿＿＿＿＿＿＿＿＿＿＿＿＿＿＿＿＿＿＿＿＿＿＿＿＿＿＿＿＿＿＿＿＿

＿＿＿＿＿＿＿＿＿＿＿＿＿＿＿＿＿＿＿＿＿＿＿＿＿＿＿＿＿＿＿＿＿＿＿

＿＿＿＿＿＿＿＿＿＿＿＿＿＿＿＿＿＿＿＿＿＿＿＿＿＿＿＿＿＿＿＿＿＿＿

COLUMN

薬が残ってしまった理由とは？

処方された薬が使い切れずに手元に残ってしまうことは多くの人が経験しています．不要になった薬は，その後どうなるのでしょうか．処方薬は，医師が患者の状態に対して必要と判断した薬ですから，手元に残ったとしても，自己判断で使用したり，他の人が使用することは勧められません．多くの場合，しばらく手元に置かれたあと，使用されないままゴミとして捨てられているのではないでしょうか．20年以上前から米国などで行われている"ブラウンバッグ運動"では，患者の手元にある不要な薬剤を薬局で積極的に回収しています．薬局が回収の窓口となることで，環境に配慮した廃棄が可能となりますが，利点はそれだけではありません．残った薬の状況を薬剤師が評価することで，患者の治療上の問題点を発見し，解決策を患者や医師に提案する機会が増えました．薬剤師が患者の身体機能やライフスタイルを考慮した処方設計を医師に提案することは，患者にとっても環境にとってもメリットがあるといえます．

（亀井美和子）

Chapter 4

Targeted Cancer Therapies

4・1 Reading

> 近年，がん治療の画期的な薬が登場した．がん細胞に特異的に発現する分子を標的とする標的がん治療薬である．標的がん治療薬は分子標的薬ともよばれ，その開発に世界中の製薬会社や研究機関が力を注いでいる．この章では，標的がん治療および分子標的薬（低分子医薬品およびモノクローナル抗体）の特徴を概説する．

What are targeted cancer therapies?

Targeted cancer therapies are drugs or other substances that block the growth and spread of cancer by interfering with specific molecules involved in tumor growth and progression. Because scientists often call these molecules "molecular targets," targeted cancer therapies are sometimes called "molecularly targeted drugs," "molecularly targeted therapies," or other similar names. By focusing on molecular and cellular changes that are specific to cancer, targeted cancer therapies may be more effective than other types of treatment, including chemotherapy and radiotherapy, and less harmful to normal cells.

Many targeted cancer therapies have been approved by the U.S. Food and Drug Administration (FDA) for the treatment of specific types of cancer. Others are being studied in clinical trials (research studies with people), and many more are in preclinical testing (research studies with animals).

Targeted cancer therapies are being studied for use alone, in combination with other targeted therapies, and in combination with other

progression 進行, 発達
molecular target 分子標的

chemotherapy 化学療法
radiotherapy 放射線療法

clinical trial 治験, 臨床試験
preclinical test 前臨床試験

cancer treatments, such as chemotherapy.

How do targeted cancer therapies work?

Targeted cancer therapies interfere with cancer cell division (proliferation) and spread in different ways. Many of these therapies focus on proteins that are involved in cell signaling pathways, which form a complex communication system that governs basic cellular functions and activities, such as cell division, cell movement, cell responses to specific external stimuli, and even cell death. By blocking signals that tell cancer cells to grow and divide uncontrollably, targeted cancer therapies can help stop cancer progression and may induce cancer cell death through a process known as apoptosis. Other targeted therapies can cause cancer cell death directly, by specifically inducing apoptosis, or indirectly, by stimulating the immune system to recognize and destroy cancer cells and/or by delivering toxic substances directly to the cancer cells.

The development of targeted therapies, therefore, requires the identification of good targets—that is, targets that are known to play a key role in cancer cell growth and survival. (It is for this reason that targeted therapies are often referred to as the product of "rational drug design.")

How are targeted therapies developed?

Once a target has been identified, a therapy must be developed. Most targeted therapies are either small-molecule drugs or monoclonal antibodies. Small-molecule drugs are typically able to diffuse into cells and can act on targets that are found inside the cell. Most monoclonal antibodies cannot penetrate the cell's plasma membrane and are directed against targets that are outside cells or on the cell surface.

Candidates for small-molecule drugs are usually identified in studies

---

proliferation 増殖

signaling pathway 情報伝達系

induce 誘発する

apoptosis アポトーシス〈プログラムされた細胞死〉↔ネクローシス

monoclonal antibody モノクローナル抗体

penetrate 透過する

plasma membrane 原形質膜, 細胞膜

known as drug screens—laboratory tests that look at the effects of thousands of test compounds on a specific target. The best candidates are then chemically modified to produce numerous closely related versions, and these are tested to identify the most effective and specific drugs.

Monoclonal antibodies, by contrast, are prepared first by immunizing animals (typically mice) with purified target molecules. The immunized animals will make many different types of antibodies against the target. Next, spleen cells, each of which makes only one type of antibody, are collected from the immunized animals and fused with myeloma cells. Cloning of these fused cells generates cultures of cells that produce large amounts of a single type of antibody, known as a monoclonal antibody. These antibodies are then tested to find the ones that react best with the target.

Before they can be used in humans, monoclonal antibodies are "humanized" by replacing as much of the animal portion of the antibody as possible with human portions. This is done through genetic engineering. Humanizing is necessary to prevent the human immune system from recognizing the monoclonal antibody as "foreign" and destroying it before it has a chance to interact with and inactivate its target molecule.

出 典：*Targeted Cancer Therapies*, National Cancer Institute at the National Institutes of Health のウェブサイト〔http://www.cancer.gov/cancertopics/factsheet/Therapy/targeted（2015 年 1 月現在）〕より転載.

4・2 Comprehension Questions
Answer the following questions in English.

1. What are the merits of targeted cancer therapies compared to other types of treatment?

   _____

2. What is the process known as apoptosis?

   _____

3. Where are the targets of small-molecule drugs and monoclonal antibodies located?

   _____

4. How are candidates for small-molecule drugs usually identified?

   _____

5. Why is humanizing necessary for the monoclonal antibody?

   _____

4・3 Grammar

Correct each sentence that is grammatically (or stylistically) wrong.
Target ➤ Adjective

1. We performed a double-blind, randomized comparison of 3 fluids for initial resuscitation of Vietnamese children with dengue shock syndrome.
2. Noroviruses are the most common pathogens in diarrhea due to foodborne infection, and poultry is associated with a highest proportion of deaths (19%).
3. IVF procedures, which are defined as procedures in which eggs and sperm are manipulated with the purpose of establishing a pregnancy, represent the overwhelming majority of procedures for assisted reproduct technology.
4. Diarrhea is generally defined as the passage of three or more unforming stools per day, often in addition to other enteric symptoms, or the passage of more than 250 g of unforming stool per day.
5. Noroviruses are particularly common in closing populations such as cruise ships, nursing homes, dormitories, and hospitals.

IVF　*in vitro* fertilization　（体外受精）

4・4 Medical Vocabulary
▶ 治療薬・治療法の名称と略語 (1)

Match each of the following words with its abbreviation below and then translate the word into Japanese.

1. carbamazepine　(　)　_____
2. erythropoietin　(　)　_____
3. methotrexate　(　)　_____
4. selective serotonin reuptake inhibitor

    (　)　_____
5. phenobarbital　(　)　_____
6. levofloxacin　(　)　_____
7. phenytoin　(　)　_____
8. urokinase　(　)　_____

a. PB
b. PHT
c. CBZ
d. SSRI
e. EPO
f. UK
g. MTX
h. LVFX

4・5 Writing
▶ **Presentation on your home town/country/culture**
Introduce your home town/country/culture to classmates.

Let me introduce _____

_____

_____

_____

_____

_____

_____

_____

COLUMN

分子標的薬 ── がん細胞と正常細胞の違いからがん細胞を狙い撃ち

　従来の多くの薬剤もその作用機序を探ると，もちろん何らかの標的分子をもつが，分子標的治療は創薬や治療法設計の段階から分子レベルの標的を定めている点で異なる．一般に，抗がん剤の多くは，がん細胞だけでなく正常細胞も攻撃してしまうので，重い有害反応が問題となることも少なくない．一方，がん細胞がもつ特有の物質の働きのみを抑えることができれば，有害反応の少ないがん治療薬になるはずとの考えから開発されたのが，分子標的薬である．

　慢性骨髄性白血病において染色体の異常が生じ，それによりつくられる酵素チロシンキナーゼ Bcr-Abl の ATP 結合部位に結合して阻害することで抗がん作用を示すとして，分子標的薬のイマチニブメシル酸塩が開発された．

　近年，コンピューターとゲノム医学の進歩により，標的分子発見後の分子標的薬の創薬期間が短縮化される傾向にある．これらは多くの薬学的な知見や高度な知識や技術の集約ではあるが，これでも治療効果や有害反応の問題は完全に解決できるものではない．今後も，治療効果がより高く，有害反応がより少ない新薬や治療法の開発は重要な課題である．

（川崎郁勇）

イマチニブメシル酸塩

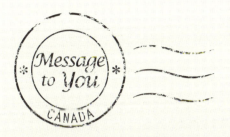

Pharmacy Practice and Education in Alberta

Hello to those students studying pharmacy in Japan!

You are in a very enviable position as you prepare to become a competent and trusted health care provider within the pharmacy profession. As a pharmacist and a very accessible health professional, you have the opportunity to play a key role in the health of your patients through a broad range of services. I encourage each of you to take up that role.

The following is a brief description of the changes in pharmacy practice in Alberta and important components of the curriculum which prepare students to support changes in practice to advance patient care. The experiences that have informed my perspective are those of one the pharmacy faculty members who have had the wonderful opportunity to coordinate the clinical placements for pharmacy students across Alberta.

As posted on the Alberta Pharmacists' Association web page message to the Public, "On July 1, 2012, a new Pharmacy Services Framework, jointly developed by the Alberta Pharmacists' Association and the Government of Alberta, came into effect. It further supports pharmacists' active role in advancing Albertans' health. Pharmacists have a key role to play in the health of Albertans and offer a broad range of services to ensure the best health outcomes for their patients. The new framework will improve patient health care access and increase efficiencies in health care delivery." This framework for pharmacy services is consistent with the Alberta College of Pharmacists' Standards of Practice implemented in 2007 within the Health Professions Act of Alberta.

Pharmacists are now reimbursed by the government for authorizing renewal of prescription medications, prescribing medications in an emergency, provision of an annual care plan or medication review for patients, refusal to fill a prescription and trial prescriptions. Pharmacists can also obtain authorization to administer a product by injection and authorization for additional prescribing authority to prescribe at initial access or manage ongoing therapy.

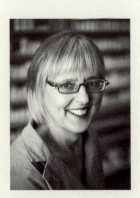

The pharmacy curriculum has also changed and students have been a key contributor to the implementation of new services. Currently the pharmacy curriculum is a 1+4 model but will be changing to a 2+4 year model in 2017 to lengthen the clinical placements consistent with the standards for the

Doctor of Pharmacy Degree. Examples of key components of the pharmacy curriculum which have helped prepare students for practice are the inclusion of direct patient care experiences in pharmacy practice in first and second year, patient simulation activities and communication skills in the pharmacy practice labs in each of the first three years, clinical modules integrating the pharmaceutical and clinical sciences, evidence based medicine and literature evaluation skills and interprofessional team building activities. In Alberta, practicing pharmacists from community and institutional practice and primary care clinics are appointed as preceptor faculty to supervise students during the clinical placements. The faculty also supports the pharmacists in the development of preceptorship skills to enhance the learning experiences in the practice setting. My closing comments are suggestions for preparing for the future roles of your profession, to be active participants and change agents. The preparation starts in the classroom and extends to your clinical placements, your work experiences and your opportunities as a volunteer and member or your community.

1. Keep in the forefront, your passion for helping your patient and for helping the patient become a good manager of their medications and health. It is a partnership. Your caring nature, your determination and enthusiasm alone can help others.
2. Explore what it means to be a professional and engage in professional relationships with your patients, peers and other health care providers. Consider professionalism as the ability to negotiate the expectations that others have of you as a pharmacist and the ability to meet those expectations. Help others realize how you can assist with their health outcomes.
3. Recognize the uncertainty in which clinical decision making is embedded. Professional judgment or critical thinking involves the integration of the best evidence, your patient's concerns and goals, additional knowledge of your patient's situation, your prior experiences, an awareness of your personal values and preferences which inform your decisions and where possible the perspectives of other members of the health care team. Ensure you collaborate and follow-up with your patients to monitor the outcome of your care.
4. Support the creation of roles for pharmacy technicians and work collaboratively in the provision of patient care.
5. Obtain work experience while a student to further develop skills initiated in the curriculum. Where possible work in a pharmacy setting or become a volunteer to help serve others to make a difference in the quality of their life. Understanding what that means for others will assist you as a pharmacist and citizen.
6. Learn from every patient and every patient care experience. Critical reflection on one's experience is necessary to guide your practice across your career.
7. Ask questions. It is important to understand the history of pharmacy practice and to

explore the feasibility of an alternate approach.
8. Collaborate with practicing pharmacists to engage in new approaches to meet the needs of your patients. Together you are the future of pharmacy practice.
9. Share in responsibility for developing the necessary competencies for the future delivery of patient care.
10. Consider how to include health promotion activities in your practice. Be aware of the determinants of health that impact your community. Become an active member of your community.

Enjoy the evolution of your practice one patient at a time and one physician or health care provider at a time. Create teams and build a community of care enhancing the patient's access to valuable services. You have selected a wonderful profession and career.

Best regards,

Cheryl Cox, BSP, MBA
Faculty of Pharmacy and Pharmaceutical Sciences
University of Alberta

Chapter 5

Insulin

5・1 Reading

> インスリンによる血中グルコース濃度の調節は，糖尿病患者にとって死活問題である．遺伝子組換え技術によってヒトインスリンが生産されるようになり，注射後すぐにその効果が現れるものや，効果が持続するように工夫された製剤も開発されている．極細の注射針やα-GI とよばれる薬も開発され，糖尿病患者の QOL は大きく向上した．

QOL　生活の質
（quality of life）

Track 5

hormone　ホルモン
secrete　分泌する
beta cell　β細胞
pancreas　膵臓
diabetes　糖尿病
inject　注射する
adequately　適切に

　A hormone secreted by the beta cells of the pancreas helps move glucose from the blood into body cells for energy. People with Type 1 diabetes lose the ability to produce insulin and must inject it. Some people with Type 2 diabetes also need to inject insulin because the insulin that is produced by their pancreas does not adequately lower their blood glucose level.

　Scientists discovered insulin in the early 1920's and found that it could be used to successfully treat diabetes. Since then, a variety of insulins have been developed to meet the different needs of people with diabetes.

　In the past, all commercially available insulin came from the pancreases of cows or pigs. Pork and beef insulins are similar to human insulin, differing only in one or a few amino acids (protein building blocks).

elicit　誘発する
allergic response　アレルギー反応

However, even a slight difference is enough to elicit an allergic response in some people. To overcome this problem, researchers looked for ways to make insulin that would more closely resemble human insulin.

　Since the early 1980's, two methods have been used to make human insulin from nonhuman sources. One method involves the use of enzymes to convert pork insulin into human insulin by altering the one amino acid that is different. The second and more widely used method uses recombinant DNA technology. In this process, bacteria or yeast cells are genetically altered to produce human insulin in large amounts. Human insulin produced by genetic engineering is purer than other forms of insulin because it is not combined with other proteins that can also trigger allergic responses. Pork and beef insulin are no longer being sold in the United States.

One of the latest advances in insulin therapy is the development of insulin analogs. There are now two types of insulin analogs on the market: rapid-acting and long-acting. Rapid-acting analogs are modified forms of human insulin that have been altered in such a way that the molecules do not clump together the way Regular insulin molecules do. This allows them to be absorbed much more quickly into the bloodstream and to begin working, peak, and break down more quickly than Regular insulin. The first rapid-acting analog to come on the market was lispro (brand name Humalog) by Eli Lilly and Company, which was approved in 1996. A second rapid-acting insulin analog, aspart (NovoLog), made by Novo Nordisk, was approved in 2000, and a third, glulisine (Apidra), made by Sanofi-aventis, was approved in 2004.

The long-acting insulin analogs are glargine (Lantus), made by Sanofi-aventis and approved in 2000, and detemir (Levemir), made by Novo Nordisk and approved in 2005. These analogs are designed to be absorbed very slowly into the bloodstream, so that their effects last for 24 hours without peaking.

All insulin regimens are made up of some combination of these different types of insulin. Some people can effectively manage their blood glucose levels with one or two injections of premixed insulin per day. These people must inject at specific times of the day, and also eat their meals at specific times. The shorter-acting insulin covers mealtimes and the longer-acting insulin maintains a steady amount of insulin in the bloodstream between meals. Some people with Type 2 diabetes manage their blood glucose levels by combining diabetes pills with one injection of longer-acting insulin in the evening or at bedtime.

 Other people inject insulin several times a day, a practice that allows greater flexibility in the timing of their meals. Multiple injection regimens generally involve taking a shot of short-acting insulin before each meal, in combination with one or two injections of longer-acting insulin in the morning or at bedtime. When Regular insulin is injected before meals, a person must wait 30 to 60 minutes before eating. When lispro is used, no waiting is generally required before eating.

出　典：*Insulin*, Diabetes Self-Management のウェブサイト〔http://www.diabetesselfmanagement.com/diabetes-resources/definitions/insulin/?print=0（2015年1月現在）〕より転載．Copyright © 2014 Madavor Media, LLC. All rights reserved.

5・2　Comprehension Questions
Answer the following questions in English.

1. Why are people with diabetes required to take insulin artificially?

　_____

2. Why are beef or pork insulin not sold in the United States?

　_____

3. How many kinds of insulin analogs have been developed?

　_____

4. What is the biochemical difference between Regular insulin and insulin analogs?

　_____

5. Explain the benefit of the rapid-acting insulin analogs for people with diabetes.

　_____

5・3　Grammar
Choose the correct answer that best fits the sentence.
Target ➤ Verb

1. Manufacturers and distributors of dietary supplements are prohibited (　　) products that are adulterated or misbranded.
    a. market　　　b. to market　　　c. marketing　　　d. from marketing

2. Rabies is a zoonotic disease, a disease that (　　) to humans from animals, that is caused by a virus.
    a. is transmitted　　b. transmits　　c. was transmitted　　d. has transmitted

3. Added color (　　) a kind of code that allows us to identify products on sight, like candy flavors, medicine dosages, and left or right contact lenses.
    a. serves　　　b. to serve　　　c. serves as　　　d. served

4. Worldwide, there are certain risk factors that (　　) some more likely to get depression than others.
    a. make　　　b. get　　　c. let　　　d. have

5. Moreover, the extension of life expectancy and the ageing of the general populations in both developed and developing countries are likely to (　　) the prevalence of many chronic and progressive physical and mental conditions including neurological disorders.
    a. rise　　　b. increase　　　c. arise　　　d. boost

adulterate　不純物を混ぜて質を落とす
rabies　狂犬病
zoonotic　人畜共通感染症の

neurological disorder　神経障害(疾患)

5・4 Medical Vocabulary
▶ 治療薬・治療法の名称と略語 (2)

Match each of the following words with its abbreviation below and then translate the word into Japanese.

1. angiotensin receptor blocker
　　　　　　　　　(　) _____
2. antimetabolite　　(　) _____
3. angiotensin-converting enzyme inhibitor
　　　　　　　　　(　) _____
4. propylthiouracil　(　) _____
5. acyclovir　　　　(　) _____
6. nitroglycerin　　(　) _____
7. oral contraceptive　(　) _____
8. disease-modifying antirheumatic drug
　　　　　　　　　(　) _____

　a. ACEI　　　　　　　e. AM
　b. ACV　　　　　　　f. OC
　c. ARB　　　　　　　g. PTU
　d. DMARD　　　　　h. NTG

5・5 Writing

▶ Explaining categories

The reading passage shows a good example of explaining "categories." Arrange the order of words and punctuation marks in the parentheses and make a sentence explaining "categories."

1. There are (and, phagocytes, of, types, :, two, leukocytes, lymphocytes).

___

2. Medicines act in a variety of ways. Some can cure an illness by killing germs such as bacteria and viruses. Others (missing, vitamins, as, replace, substances, hormones, such).

___

COLUMN

インスリン製剤に注目！──超速効型と持効型の工夫を解き明かそう

　糖尿病の治療に使用されるインスリンには"超速効型"や"持効型"の製剤がある．これらの製剤では，皮下投与後，どのような機序によって効果を速やかに発現したり，持続したりするのだろうか？　ヒトと同じアミノ酸配列のインスリンは製剤中で六量体を形成している．そのため皮下投与したインスリンは，六量体から二量体を経て単量体になった後，毛細血管に吸収され作用を発現する．超速効型では，ヒトインスリンのアミノ酸配列を一部置換し，作用には影響を及ぼさず，インスリン分子間の反発を強め，単量体になりやすくすることにより，皮下組織から毛細血管への吸収を速めた．一方，持効型は，皮下でいったん析出して徐々に溶解したり，分子間の親和性を高めて単量体になるのを遅らせたり，血中でアルブミンと結合するような化学修飾を行った．このように，インスリン製剤には，物理化学における分子間相互作用や溶解度，生物化学における遺伝子組換え，薬物動態学における吸収とタンパク質結合など，多くの薬学的な知見が集約されている．ぜひ，各製剤の工夫について調べ，科学技術の応用を確認してみよう．　　　　（中村明弘）

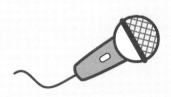
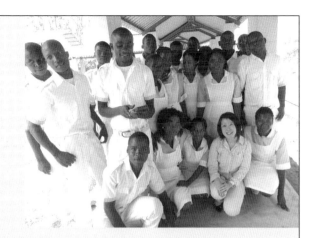

My Path to JICA

Eric: Hello, Chizuko. First, thank you for agreeing to be interviewed. We appreciate it. Can you tell us about your educational background?

Chizuko: Hello, Eric. It is my pleasure. I went to junior high & high school at Kamakura Jyogakuin girls junior and high school where I specialized in science and mathematics.

For my undergraduate studies I went to Tokyo University of Pharmacy and Life Sciences (TUPLS), as you well know. And for my graduate studies, I also studied at TUPLS where I studied in the clinical pharmaceutical program.

Eric: After you graduated, what was your first job?

Chizuko: After graduating, I started to work at St. Marianna University School of Medicine Hospital as a clinical pharmacist. I worked in the department of chemotherapy.

Eric: Why did you decide to become that kind of pharmacist?

Chizuko: During my hospital practice for six months, in my graduate studies, I learned many skills about how to care for patients as a clinical pharmacist. After I graduated, I wanted to learn even more about clinical treatment and to get better skills as a member of a patient care team, so I decided to work at a university hospital to learn many things.

Eric: You are now working for JICA. Why?

Chizuko: When I was a junior high student, I watched a TV program about the volunteer work of JICA. The volunteer who worked in some countries of Asia would help the local people to construct a well in their village. At that time, I thought that working in other countries is interesting.

Also, during and after high school, I did homestays and studied English in Canada and, during my university days, I studied English in the U.S. many times. And luckily, when I was a third-year student pharmacist and in grad school, I also had chances to study clinical pharmacy at UCSF. On top of that, I traveled a lot all over the world during my university days and made many friends, and I learned a lot about the medical situations of developing countries.

All these experiences in foreign countries inspired and stimulated me strongly to work outside of Japan as a pharmacist, especially in developing countries.

JICA is the biggest association in Japan to work internationally not only in Japan but also in foreign countries and some projects matched my desire. So I decided to work for JICA in order to help many people and experience many things.

Eric: And from January, 2014, you have been in Mozambique. How have you liked Mozambique so far?

Chizuko: Mozambique is not rich, but is a very nice country, because they have a wealth of nature, lovely beaches, and lots of delicious foods. In regard to the food, there is their traditional cuisine and Portuguese or other foreign cuisines. I love to learn how to cook these cuisines. And more, the people are gentle, kind, cheerful, and they love to dance and make music. Where I live, the people dance, sing, and drink almost all night every weekend. It is so fun! I live in Quelimane, which is a large city in Mozambique. It is very nice here. There are many sightseeing spots, for example, beautiful beaches, rich nature, and the city is famous for "Zambezia Chicken". This dish is very tasty and the most delicious chicken in all of Mozambique.

Eric: We are almost finished. Can you please share a message to the student pharmacists of Japan?

Chizuko: Sure. To be a pharmacist is a job that has many opportunities and possibilities. First, we have to think about patient care, but the methods are varied. During your life in your university, learn, try, ask and feel many things. Don't be afraid of failure. Find your dream and get it. Good luck!

Eric: Thank you, Chizuko. Best of luck helping the people of Mozambique and growing as a pharmacist!

Chapter 6

The Immune System

6・1 Reading

> 生体は常にさまざまな病原体と戦っている．免疫細胞には役割分担がある．侵略者を見つける，敵襲来の情報を伝達する，攻撃開始を命令する，武器を作る，攻撃する，攻撃の始まりや終わりを告げるなど，免疫細胞のそれぞれが独自の役割をもって敵と戦う．この精密で合理的なヒト免疫系のチームプレーをみてみよう．

Track 6

The human immune system is a complex network of cells and organs that evolved to fight off infectious microbes. Much of the immune system's work is carried out by an army of various specialized cells, each type designed to fight disease in a particular way. The invading microbes first run into the vanguard of this army, which includes white blood cells called macrophages (literally, "big eaters"). The macrophages engulf as many of the microbes as they can.

macrophage　マクロファージ，大食細胞

Antigens sound the alarm

How do the macrophages recognize the microbes? All cells and microbes wear a "uniform" made up of molecules that cover their surfaces. Each human cell displays unique marker molecules unique to you. Microbes display different marker molecules unique to them. The macrophages and other cells of your immune system use these markers to distinguish among the cells that are part of your body, harmless bacteria that reside in your body, and harmful invading microbes that need to be destroyed.

marker molecule
マーカー分子

The molecules on a microbe that identify it as foreign and stimulate the immune system to attack it are called "antigens." Every microbe carries its own unique set of antigens, which are central to creating vaccines.

Macrophages digest most parts of the microbes but save the antigens and carry them back to the lymph nodes, bean-sized organs scattered throughout your body where immune system cells congregate. In these nodes, macrophages sound the alarm by "regurgitating" the antigens, displaying them on their surfaces so other cells, such as specialized defensive white blood cells called lymphocytes, can recognize them.

Lymphocytes take over

There are two major kinds of lymphocytes, T cells and B cells, and they do their own jobs in fighting off infection. T cells function either offensively or defensively. The offensive T cells don't attack the microbe directly, but they use chemical weapons to eliminate the human cells that have already been infected. Because they have been "programmed" by their exposure to the microbe's antigen, these cytotoxic T cells, also called killer T cells, can "sense" diseased cells that are harboring the microbe. The killer T cells latch onto these cells and release chemicals that destroy the infected cells and the microbes inside.

The defensive T cells, also called helper T cells, defend the body by secreting chemical signals that direct the activity of other immune system cells. Helper T cells assist in activating killer T cells, and helper T cells also stimulate and work closely with B cells. The work done by T cells is called the cellular or cell-mediated immune response.

B cells make and secrete extremely important molecular weapons called antibodies. Antibodies usually work by first grabbing onto the microbe's antigen, and then sticking to and coating the microbe. Antibodies and antigens fit together like pieces of a jigsaw puzzle—if their shapes are compatible, they bind to each other.

Each antibody can usually fit with only one antigen. The immune system keeps a supply of millions and possibly billions of different antibodies on hand to be prepared for any foreign invader. It does this by constantly creating millions of new B cells. About 50 million B cells
5 circulate in each teaspoonful of human blood, and almost every B cell produces a unique antibody that it displays on its surface.

When these B cells come into contact with their matching microbial antigen, they are stimulated to divide into many larger cells, called plasma cells, which secrete mass quantities of antibodies to bind to the microbe.

plasma cell　形質細胞

Antibodies in action

10　The antibodies secreted by B cells circulate throughout the human body and attack the microbes that have not yet infected any cells but are lurking in the blood or the spaces between cells. When antibodies gather on the surface of a microbe, it becomes unable to function. Antibodies
15 signal macrophages and other defensive cells to come eat the microbe. Antibodies also work with other defensive molecules that circulate in the blood, called complement proteins, to destroy microbes.

complement protein
補体タンパク質

When T cells and antibodies begin to eliminate the microbe faster than it can reproduce, the immune system finally has the upper hand.
20 Gradually, the virus disappears from the body.

出典：*Vaccines*, The National Institute of Allergy and Infectious Diseases のウェブサイト
〔http://www.niaid.nih.gov/topics/vaccines/understanding/Pages/howWork.aspx（2015 年 1 月現在）〕より転載.

6・2　Comprehension Questions
Based on the reading passage, circle T (true) or F (false) for each statement.

1. The immune system's work is independently carried out by each of the specialized cells.　　　　　　　　　　　　　　　　　　　(T , F)
2. The cells of the human immune system use marker molecules unique to your body to distinguish invading foreign cells.　　　　　　(T , F)

3. For creating vaccines, the molecules unique to a microbe called antigens are important. (T , F)
4. While defensive T cells use chemicals to destroy harmful cells, killer T cells latch onto and eat them. (T , F)
5. An antibody comes and sticks to the most active antigen near at hand, binding to each other. (T , F)

6・3 Grammar

Rewrite the word(s) in the parentheses of numbers 1, 3, 4, and 5 in an appropriate manner. And rewrite the words in the parentheses of number 2 into an infinitive phrase.

Target ➤ Infinitive

1. The FDA works with other government agencies and private sector organizations to help (reducing) the risk of tampering or other malicious, criminal, or terrorist actions on the food and cosmetic supply.
2. The Mental Health Gap Action Programme (mhGAP) has produced evidence-based guidelines for non-specialists to enable them (in identification and management of mental health priority conditions).
3. A novel protein nanoparticle has shown (be) effective at getting the immune system to attack the most lethal species of malaria parasite, *Plasmodium falciparum*.
4. The purpose of this report is to raise awareness of dementia as a public health priority, to articulate a public health approach and (advocating) for action at international and national levels.
5. After virus incubation for 4–10 days, an infected mosquito is capable (to transmit) the virus for the rest of its life.

mhGAP　世界精神保健アクションプログラム

6・4 Medical Vocabulary
▶ 医薬品開発関連の用語と略語 (1)

Match each of the following abbreviated words with its meaning below and then translate the word into Japanese.

1. CRC   ( ) _____
2. CRO   ( ) _____
3. DEM   ( ) _____
4. GMP   ( ) _____
5. DBT   ( ) _____
6. DI   ( ) _____
7. DSU   ( ) _____
8. GCP   ( ) _____

a. double blind test
b. contract research organization
c. drug information
d. clinical research coordinator
e. good clinical practice
f. good manufacturing practice
g. drug event monitoring
h. drug safety update

6・5 Writing
▶ **Explaining a process/procedure**

You are head of a student union, and need to explain how to reserve a classroom for club activities. Explain the procedures of your university in English.

Hi, everyone, I will tell you how to reserve a classroom for club activities at this university. First,

---

COLUMN

免疫は"諸刃の剣"

1798年，Edward Jennerは種痘によって天然痘を防ぐことができることを発見し，ワクチンを用いる予防接種の考え方が生まれました．感染免疫学の幕開けです．これを契機に病原体に対する予防接種がつぎつぎと開発され，感染症治療が著しく変貌してきました．予防接種は病原体に対する二次応答が早く強く起きることを応用したものです．この一連の反応には，免疫に関わるさまざまな臓器，組織，細胞，分子が関与しています．好中球やマクロファージが病原体を捕捉し殺菌し，その情報を抗原提示細胞の力を借りてTリンパ球に伝え，サイトカインや傷害分子を分泌し，Bリンパ球は抗体を産生します．

一方で，免疫系はアレルギー疾患，自己免疫疾患など，生体にとって不都合な反応をひき起こすことから，諸刃の剣（a double-edged sword）といわれています．生体の恒常性は，神経系，内分泌系，免疫系，さらには常在微生物叢によって制御されています．不都合な免疫反応を軽減するために，これらの軸のバランスを制御する方法の開発が急がれています．

（大野尚仁）

Chapter 7

Low-Fat Diet Not a Cure-All

7・1 Reading

脂肪を控える食事は，一般的に健康によいと思われている．心臓病や癌予防にどの程度効果があるか，1993年に約5万人の女性で8年間に及ぶ大規模な調査が行われた．効果はまったくないという結果に，研究方法について専門家から多くの疑問点が提示され，研究の評価にはいまだ意見が分かれている．仮説から結果を得るまでどのような研究方法で検証したか，何が説得力を得るために必要なのか，さまざまな観点から考えてみる必要があるだろう．

Women's Health Initiative (WHI)　女性健康イニシアティブ〈1991年米国国立衛生研究所 (NIH) により設立された，更年期以降の米国女性のさまざまな疾患原因を研究する機関〉

Dietary Modification Trial　食事療法臨床試験

Results from the large, long Women's Health Initiative Dietary Modification Trial shows no effect on heart disease, breast cancer, colorectal cancer, or weight.

The trial and its findings

The Women's Health Initiative Dietary Modification Trial was started back in 1993, at a time when dietary fat was seen as a dietary evil and the low-fat diet was thought to be a straightforward route to preventing heart disease, some cancers, and the epidemic of obesity that was beginning to

sweep　圧倒する，夢中にさせる

the National Heart, Lung, and Blood Institute　国立心肺血液研究所 (NHI)〈米国立衛生研究所の20ある研究所の一つ〉

sweep the country. With funding from the National Heart, Lung, and Blood Institute, researchers recruited almost 50,000 women between the ages of 50 and 79 years. Of these, 19,541 were randomly assigned to follow a low-fat diet. Their goal was to lower their fat intake from almost 38% of calories to 20%. They were helped in this effort by a series of individual and group counseling sessions. Another 29,294 women were randomly assigned to continue their usual diets, and were given just

generic　包括的な，全体的な

generic diet-related educational materials.

After eight years, the researchers looked at how many (and what percentage) of women in each group had developed breast cancer or colorectal cancer. They tallied up heart attacks, strokes, and other forms of heart disease. They also looked at things like weight gain or loss, cholesterol levels, and other measures of health.

The results, published in the *Journal of the American Medical Association*, showed no benefits for a low-fat diet. Women assigned to this eating strategy did not appear to gain protection against breast cancer, colorectal cancer, or cardiovascular disease. And after eight years, their weights were generally the same as those of women following their usual diets.

Limitations of the study

Some nutrition experts say that the WHI Dietary Modification Trial doesn't really lay to rest the low-fat hypothesis because the women in the study only modestly lowered their fat, from 38% to 29%. Had they reached the trial's target of 20%, benefits from the low-fat approach may have become more apparent, these nutritionists suggest.

It is possible that the participants in the low-fat group may have actually overstated how much they reduced their fat intake. This has happened in other studies, as shown by comparisons between self-reported changes and biochemical measures of dietary change. Significant reductions in fat intake are usually reflected in a decrease in HDL (good) cholesterol and an increase in triglycerides. Yet in the WHI trial, there were no differences in blood levels of HDL cholesterol or triglycerides between the low-fat and usual diet groups. This casts doubt on the degree of fat reduction achieved in this study.

Two other limitations of the trial are the study population and duration. The trial included women who were aged 50 to 79 years at the beginning

chronic 慢性の

of the trial. By this time in life, it may be too late for changes in diet to reduce risks of cancer and other chronic conditions. In addition, it takes years for the effects of dietary change to be seen, and so it is possible that eight years wasn't enough time to see the true impact of a low-fat diet.

The debate will likely continue as to why the WHI observed little benefit for a low-fat diet. Was it because reducing the intake of dietary fat truly has little benefit? Was it because the women in the trial didn't lower fat intake enough? Or had the study focused on a younger population, or lasted longer, would it have revealed a benefit?

In any case, the dietary intervention didn't work, even though the WHI trial was, by far, the most expensive study of diet ever conducted (costing many hundreds of millions of dollars) and even though the women in the low-fat group received intensive dietary counseling from some of the best nutritionists and dietitians in the country.

出 典: *Low-Fat Diet Not a Cure-All*, Harvard School of Public Health のホームページ〔http://www.hsph.harvard.edu/nutritionsource/low-fat/（2015年1月現在）〕より転載.

7・2 Comprehension Questions

1. Based on the reading passage, circle T (true) or F (false) for each statement.

（1）The participants of the study could be too old to get the true effects of a dietary change. (T , F)

（2）The subjects of the low-fat group showed some decrease in good cholesterol levels and increases in triglycerides, which is considered to result from the reduction of fat intake. (T , F)

（3）Some nutritionists are skeptical of the study because the subjects of the study did not lower their fat intake enough to get the benefits. (T , F)

（4）The study had huge financial support from a national organization.

（5）All participants of the study directly received some dietary advice from experts during the study. (T , F)

（6）According to some critics, the 8-year study was not long enough to reveal the effects of the diet. (T , F)

2. What other factors do you think the study needs to look at?
e.g. Mediterranean diet, genetic information, life styles (smoking habit, sedentary life, etc.)

7・3 Grammar

Rewrite the word(s) in the parentheses to help make a proper sentence.

Target ➤ Gerund

1. An important part of mosquito control around your home is (make) sure that mosquitoes don't have a place to lay their eggs.
2. (Know) the different stages of the mosquito's life will help you prevent mosquitoes around your home and also help you choose the right pesticides for your needs, if you decide to use them.
3. You can reduce your risk of being infected with West Nile Virus by using insect repellent and (wear) protective clothing to prevent mosquito bites.
4. Shortages of drugs and biologics pose a significant public health threat, (delay), and in some cases even (deny), critically needed care for patients.
5. Early and open dialogue between FDA and manufacturers is critical to successfully (mitigate and prevent) shortages.

biologics 生物製剤

mitigate （怒り，苦痛を）和らげる

7・4 Medical Vocabulary

▶ 医薬品開発関連の用語と略語 (2)

Match each of the following words with its abbreviation below and then translate the word into Japanese.

1. post marketing surveillance ( ) _____
2. International Conference on Harmonization of Technical Requirements for Registration of Pharmaceuticals for Human Use
    ( ) _____
3. institutional review board ( ) _____
4. interview form ( ) _____
5. quality assurance ( ) _____
6. good laboratory practice ( ) _____
7. quality control ( ) _____
8. medical representative ( ) _____

a. ICH
b. IRB
c. PMS
d. GLP
e. MR
f. QC
g. QA
h. IF

7・5 Writing

▶ **Evaluating a study**

1. What other factors do you think the study in this chapter should/could have considered?

Hints❗

The study should have considered....

_____
_____
_____
_____

2. What are the strengths of the study?

Hints❗

The study is meaningful (important) because....

_____
_____
_____
_____

COLUMN

ポリフェノールとは

ポリフェノールは,分子内に複数のフェノール性ヒドロキシ基をもつ植物成分の総称で,特定保健用食品の機能成分である茶カテキンやフレンチパラドックスで話題になった赤ワインに多く含まれるレスベラトロールなどのフラボノイドがよく知られているが,その構造は多岐にわたり,5000種を超えるといわれている.ポリフェノールが健康によい食品成分として注目されるようになったのは,その強い抗酸化作用が明らかになってきたことにある.この抗酸化作用は,フェノール性ヒドロキシ基が非常に酸化されやすく,フリーラジカルに水素原子を供与してその生成を抑える機能と,複数のヒドロキシ基によって活性酸素生成の原因となる遊離の銅や鉄の捕捉(キレート形成)機能によるものと考えられている.たとえば,モルヒネはケシでしか合成されないように,多くの植物は種固有の二次代謝系をもっていることから,今後多くの植物を対象とした探索によって,さらに強い抗酸化作用をもった新規ポリフェノールが発見されることが期待される.

(平田収正)

German Pharmacy Education

Dear students,

The Japanese and Germany pharmaceutical systems have a long history of co-operation and common routes. German pharmaceutical university education is divided into basic study (first to fourth semester), main study (fifth to eighth semester) and then one year of practical education. Within this subdivision three state exams are taken. The educational system for pharmacy is a mandatory regulation for the whole country with 22 university locations. Five disciplines with close interactions and several overlapping are studied: pharmaceutical / medicinal chemistry, pharmaceutical biology, pharmaceutical technology, pharmacology and toxicology as well as clinical pharmacy. The teaching lectures are accompanied by numerous practical, seminars, and excursions. The combination of theory and practice gives great help for improved understanding and application. Although the teaching on medication is connected to various aspects in medicine, the main impact is on life science areas. The combination of different natural sciences makes this an attractive and broad field of learning. Different therapeutic aspects on patients help improve communication skills in addition to enhancing the level of knowledge in all fields of patient-oriented natural science education. It starts with some inorganic salts and goes to complex immune reactions by highly specific protein-based antibodies. The learning demands on the students are on the same conditions for basic as for applied sciences. Modern techniques and methods for highly equipped state-of-the-art laboratories have to be learned as well as the possibilities to perform preparation and analytics of medicines under field conditions. The whole value chain of drug development from target identification to lead finding and optimization with biochemical and preclinical screening to early clinical phase and the design as well as the evaluation of these clinical trials show the complex network in life sciences on the possibilities for pharmacotherapeutic interventions.

Teaching should always be connected to excellent research and thereby give students the possibility to join these laboratory facilities within their time of study. Most of the teaching is performed in German due to the law regulations, but the possibilities for foreign students to join the education or research facilities are steadily expanding. It is always worth asking for some internships or positions for PhD studies for excellent foreign students. Almost all academic research facilities are internationally oriented and provide possibilities for tremendous pharmaceutical careers. Most of the former students work in public pharmacies, but the university education opens the possibilities for the pharmaceutical industries, hospitals, military or governmental positions as well as for numerous non-pharmaceutical positions related to the health sciences and health care systems.

It is clear that a great workload and huge amount of information have to be handled within the academic years in pharmaceutical education and since the progress will never stop one has to proceed with the learning the whole life through. I have chosen pharmaceutical education for my own career due to the plentiful, variable, and fascinating aspects in natural sciences with different therapeutical perspectives. It is a great honor and pleasure for me to mention the conditions and possibilities of the pharmacy study in Germany. Take the best from your own pharmaceutical education. It is up to you what you want to give back to society. Always remember that health is one of the most important things in life and it is practically required for everything.

> Holger Stark, PhD
> Univ.-Prof. Pharmaceutical and Medicinal Chemistry
> Heinrich-Heine-Universitaet Duesseldorf
> Institut fuer Pharmazeutische and Medizinische Chemie

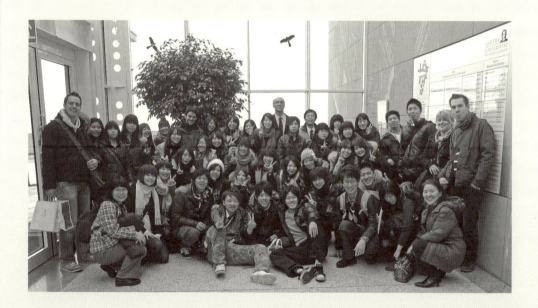

Chapter 8
Air Quality Deteriorating in Many of the World's Cities

8・1 Reading

> 2006年に米国のAl Gore元副大統領が発表した"An Inconvenient Truth (不都合な真実)"という映画は，環境汚染に対して大きな警告を発した．しかしながらその後も大気汚染は軽減されたとはいえず，さまざまなメディアで健康被害が報告されている．この章ではWHOの調査報告を読み，その文体の特徴に留意しながら内容を把握する演習を行う．このようなウェブ上の公的報告書の原文を読んで，内容を速やかに，かつ正確に理解できることは，薬学部卒業生にとって重要なことである．

deteriorate 悪化する〈ニュースや報告書のヘッドラインではbe動詞が省略されることが多い〉

Track 8

7 MAY 2014 | GENEVA — Air quality in most cities worldwide that monitor outdoor (ambient) air pollution fails to meet WHO guidelines for safe levels, putting people at additional risk of respiratory disease and other health problems.

ambient 環境の

respiratory 呼吸器官の

5　The WHO's urban air quality database covers 1600 cities across 91 countries — 500 more cities than the previous database (2011), revealing that more cities worldwide are monitoring outdoor air quality, reflecting growing recognition of air pollution's health risks.

urban 都会の，都市部の

Only 12% of the people living in cities reporting on air quality reside in
10　citics where this complies with WHO air quality guideline levels. About half of the urban population being monitored is exposed to air pollution that is at least 2.5 times higher than the levels the WHO recommends — putting those people at additional risk of serious, long-term health problems.

reside 住む

comply 応じる，従う

15　In most cities where there is enough data to compare the situation today with previous years, air pollution is getting worse. Many factors contribute to this increase, including reliance on fossil fuels such as coal fired power plants, dependence on private transport motor vehicles, inefficient use of energy in buildings, and the use of biomass for cooking and heating.

But some cities are making notable improvements — demonstrating that air quality can be improved by implementing policy measures such as banning the use of coal for "space heating" in buildings, using renewable or "clean" fuels for electricity production, and improving efficiency of motor vehicle engines.

Health risks caused by air pollution

The latest available data have prompted the WHO to call for greater awareness of health risks caused by air pollution, implementation of effective air pollution mitigation policies; and close monitoring of the situation in cities worldwide.

"Too many urban centres today are so enveloped in dirty air that their skylines are invisible," said Dr Flavia Bustreo, WHO Assistant Director-General for Family, Children and Women's Health. "Not surprisingly, this air is dangerous to breathe. So a growing number of cities and communities worldwide are striving to better meet the needs of their residents — in particular children and the elderly."

In April 2014, the WHO issued new information estimating that outdoor air pollution was responsible for the deaths of some 3.7 million people under the age of 60 in 2012. The organization also emphasised that indoor and outdoor air pollution combined are among the largest risks to health worldwide.

There are many components of air pollution, both gaseous and solid. But high concentrations of small and fine particulate pollution is particularly associated with high numbers of deaths from heart disease and stroke, as well as respiratory illnesses and cancers. Measurement of fine particulate matter of 2.5 micrometers or less in diameter (PM2.5) is considered to be the best indicator of the level of health risks from air pollution.

In high-income countries, 816 cities reported on PM2.5 levels with another 544 cities reporting on PM10, from which estimates of PM2.5 can be derived. In low- and middle-income countries, however, annual mean PM2.5 measurements could be accessed in only 70 cities; another 512 cities reported on PM10 measurements.

Measures to clean air

"We can win the fight against air pollution and reduce the number of people suffering from respiratory and heart disease, as well as lung cancer," said Dr Maria Neira, WHO Director for Public Health, Environmental and Social Determinants of Health. "Effective policies and strategies are well understood, but they need to be implemented at sufficient scale. Cities such as Copenhagen and Bogotá, for example, have

Bogotá ボゴタ〈コロンビアの首都〉

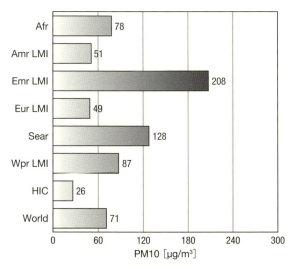

Figure PM10 levels by region, for the last available year in the period 2008-2012
The world's average PM10 levels by region range from 26 to 208 μg/m³, with a world's average of 71 μg/m³. PM10 values are regional urban population-weighted. 〔出典：*Ambient (outdoor) Air Pollution in Cities Database 2014*, World Health Organization のウェブサイト〔Public health and environment health topics; http://www.who.int/phe/health_topics/outdoorair/databases/cities/en/（2015年1月現在）〕より許可を得て転載.〕

active transport 能動輸送〈生物用語〉
dedicated network 専用ネットワーク

improved air quality by promoting 'active transport' and prioritizing dedicated networks of urban public transport, walking and cycling."

The report notes that individual cities can take local action to improve air quality and thus go against regional trends. And good air quality can go hand in hand with economic development, as indicated by some major cities in Latin America which meet, or approach, the WHO air quality guidelines.

出 典：*Air Quality Deteriorating in Many of the World's Cities*, World Health Organization のウェブサイト〔News release 7 May 2014; http://www.who.int/mediacentre/news/releases/2014/air-quality/en/（2015 年 1 月現在）〕より許可を得て転載．

8・2 Comprehension Questions

Based on the reading passage, circle T (true) or F (false) for each statement.

1. In 2011, 900 cities were covered in the WHO's urban air quality database.　　　　(T , F)
2. In 2014, there were cities which improved their air quality by implementing some measures.　　　　(T , F)
3. Air pollution was responsible for the deaths of 3.7 million young children in 2012.　　　　(T , F)
4. Fine particulate pollution is associated with diseases of the bones and glands.　　　　(T , F)
5. It is important to implement effective policies on a large scale in order to fight air pollution.　　　　(T , F)
6. High-income countries had the lowest level of PM10 in the world in the period 2008-2012.　　　　(T , F)
7. African countries marked a lower level of PM10 than that of the world average.　　　　(T , F)

8・3 Grammar

Rewrite the word(s) in the parentheses into the proper grammatical form.
Target ▶ Tense

1. By 2025, half of the world's population (live) in water-stressed areas. Re-use of wastewater, to recover water, nutrients, or energy, (become) an important strategy.
2. Japan (long battle) one of the highest suicide rates in the industrialized world. In 2012, its national rate of suicide (stand) at 18.5 deaths per 100 000 people.
3. Depression is a common mental disorder that (present) with depressed mood, loss of interest or pleasure, decreased energy, feelings of guilt or low self-worth, disturbed sleep or appetite, and poor concentration.

4. It is hoped that the report (promote) dementia as a public health and social care priority worldwide.   dementia 認知症
5. Over the past decade, a number of clinical trials (show) the effectiveness of treatment for depression across a range of resource settings.

8・4 Medical Vocabulary
▶ 入院・検査・診断に関する用語と略語 (1)

Match each of the following abbreviated words with its meaning below and then translate the word into Japanese.

1. SOAP   (   ) _____
2. VS   (   ) _____
3. BP   (   ) _____
4. HR   (   ) _____
5. P (PR) (   ) _____
6. PE   (   ) _____
7. T (BT) (   ) _____
8. R (RR) (   ) _____

a. heart rate
b. physical examination
c. blood pressure
d. subjective, objective, assessment, and plan
e. (body) temperature
f. respiratory rate
g. vital signs
h. pulse (rate)

8・5 Writing
▶ **Explaining a graph**

What can you say from the graph on page 51?

1. Compare any two areas and write a sentence about them.

_____
_____
_____
_____
_____
_____

2. Write about the mean (=average) level of PM10.

   This graph shows _____
   _____
   _____
   _____
   _____
   _____
   _____

3. Write about the highest level of PM10.

   According to this graph, _____
   _____
   _____
   _____
   _____
   _____
   _____

COLUMN

微小粒子状物質 "PM2.5"

　中国において深刻な大気汚染を招いている PM2.5 とは，大気中を浮遊する粒子状物質（SPM; suspended particulate matter）のうち，粒子径が 2.5 μm 以下のものを指す．実際には 2.5 μm の粒子を 50％ 分離できる分粒装置で採集された微粒子の集まりであり，日本では分類上 "微小微粒子物質" とよばれる．PM2.5 は，工場排煙やディーゼル車排気ガスに含まれるすすのように発生源から直接排出される一次粒子と，大気中での光化学反応などにより種々のガス成分から生成される二次粒子に分類される．SPM は呼吸器疾患などをひき起こすおそれがあり，特に PM2.5 は気管支や肺まで達し，重篤な疾患の原因となる可能性も指摘されている．そこで欧米諸国では，PM2.5 について独立項目として環境目標値が設定されており，近年偏西風により中国から飛来する PM2.5 の著しい増加が懸念される日本でも，2009 年に "1 年平均値が 15 μg/m^3 以下であり，かつ，1 日平均値が 35 μg/m^3 以下であること" とする環境基準が告示された．最近，さらに粒子径が小さい "超微小微粒子物質" の健康影響も危惧されるようになっており，これらに対する包括的な対策が望まれるところである．

（平田收正）

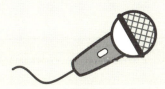
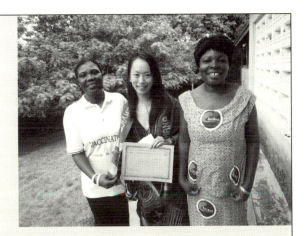

Working as a JICA Volunteer in Ghana

Today I have the honor to interview Ms. Yoko Gocho. Ms. Gocho worked as a volunteer for JICA and was sent to Ghana to work as an HIV controller. In short, she helped coordinate HIV prevention or health education projects at the community level in Ghana. Here is a brief interview I had with her.

Eric: First, thank you for agreeing to the interview.
Yoko: My pleasure, Mr. Skier.
Eric: I guess the obvious question is: were you always interested in pharmacy and English?
Yoko: Actually no. Many people misunderstand that I am originally good at English or pharmacy. To be honest, I wasn't so good at either subject.
   When I was 2nd-year student, I attended IPSF world congress for the first time and understood almost nothing. I was shocked but at the same time I realized the importance of English and pharmacy. Luckily I was able to make a lot of friends from overseas and that motivated me to study English and pharmacy more.
Eric: Interesting. So, how did you get to know about JICA?
Yoko: When I started thinking of my future career, I was looking for an opportunity to work in an international environment. Some professors who had worked at the WHO told me that there are opportunities for healthcare professionals including pharmacists to be JICA volunteers and help people in developing countries.
Eric: What were some interesting experiences while you were in Ghana?
Yoko: About a year had passed since I'd been in Ghana, and one of my colleagues (not Japanese) came up to me and said, "Hey Yoko, you gained weight, right? Congratulations!" I was so surprised and unhappy to hear that, but she looked so happy. She told me that it is good thing to be fat in Ghana. Then I was surprised again. I enjoyed local food every day and as a result, I had in fact gained weight! I learned many ideas that were taken for granted in Japan, such as thinner is better, were sometimes totally the opposite in Ghana.

Eric: That's right. In many cultures around the world, a bigger woman is better. Can you share a final message to student pharmacists in Japan?

Yoko: The chief of a village in Ghana will always help children whose parents don't have enough money to send their child to school. If anybody in a family gets sick, all the relatives or friends will help him or her to go to the hospital. I saw this behavior often when I was in Ghana and it impressed me a lot. Of course there are a lot of challenges in their daily life, yet the people in Ghana always smile and they swear they love their own country. My time in Ghana definitely enriched my entire life and I wouldn't have acquired those experiences if I hadn't gone abroad or interacted with people who have a different culture. I believe English skills are a tool to expand your world and can be a passport to meeting people who can influence your values or senses.

Eric: Thank you so much for your time, Ms. Gocho.

Yoko: My pleasure.

Chapter 9
Mental Health of Older Adults, Addressing a Growing Concern

9・1 Reading

> 精神・神経系疾患の発症には，種々の要因がある．本章では，加齢に起因する代表的な疾患である老年期うつ病と認知症に関して，WHO が情報発信しているグローバルな記述を読む．医療と福祉に関わる知見を得て，わが国の少子高齢化社会の中で直面している問題とその中で薬剤師の果たすべき社会的役割を考え，薬学生としての視野を広げよう．

Track 9

The theme of World Mental Health Day in 2013 is "Mental health and older adults".

Background

Currently, the number of people aged 60 and over is more than 800 million. Projections indicate that this figure will increase to over two billion in 2050. People aged 60 can now expect to survive an additional 18.5 to 21.6 years. Soon the world will have a higher number of older adults than children.

Older adults face special health challenges. Many of the very old lose their ability to live independently because of limited mobility, frailty or other physical or mental health problems and require some form of long-term care. Early on, in the beginning of the millennium, it became clear in the USA that about 20% of adults aged 55 and over suffer from a mental disorder.

Underlying factors of mental health problems in older adults

An important risk factor to the health and mental health of older adults,

---

mental health　精神保健, メンタルヘルス, 心の健康, 精神的健康, 精神保健衛生などいろいろな訳し方がされている

frailty　虚弱, フレイル〈frailty の訳語は従来 "加齢に伴って不可逆的に老い衰えた状態" の "虚弱" となっているが, frailty には "しかるべき介入により再び健常な状態に戻る可逆性" という意味が含まれているため, 日本老年医学会は "フレイル" の使用を表明している〉

long-term care　長期的ケア

mental disorder　精神障害

risk factor　危険因子, リスクファクター

and an important human rights issue, is elder maltreatment. WHO defines elder maltreatment as "a single or repeated act, or lack of appropriate action, occurring within any relationship where there is an expectation of trust that causes harm or distress to an older person." Elder maltreatment can lead not only to physical injuries but also to serious, sometimes long-lasting psychological consequences, including depression and anxiety.

Physical health problems in older adults

Mental health has a big impact on physical health. For example, coexisting depression in people with diabetes is associated with decreased adherence to treatment, poor metabolic control, higher complication rates, decreased quality of life, increased healthcare use and cost, increased disability and lost productivity, and increased risk of death. Conversely, people with medical conditions such as heart disease, diabetes, asthma and arthritis have higher rates of depression than those who are medically well.

Mental disorders in older adults

Dementia

Dementia is a syndrome involving deterioration in memory, thinking, behaviour and the ability to perform everyday activities such as dressing, eating, personal hygiene and toilet activities. It generally affects older people, although it is not a normal part of ageing. A report by WHO and Alzheimer Disease Association International (ADI) in 2012 suggests a crude estimated prevalence of 4.7% among people 60 years and over. Though no cure is available, much can be done for people with dementia and their caregivers. A range of pharmacological and several non-pharmacological interventions are available and can be delivered by even non-specialized health providers.

Depression

Depression is common in old age. Symptoms of older adults' depression differ only in part from early life depression. Effective psychological and pharmacological treatments exist; however, great care needs to be taken when prescribing antidepressants to this age group. Health care providers should prescribe reduced initial doses of antidepressants and finish with lower final doses. If severe, depression may lead to suicide. Comorbidity with alcohol use disorders increases the likelihood.

Other mental disorders

Stressful life events such as retirement, marital breakdown or bereavement, social isolation, financial problems, mental disorders and some chronic physical conditions are main contributing factors to substance abuse. Physiological changes associated with ageing and increased use of other medicines, especially sedatives, may make drinking in lower doses more harmful for older adults through inducing more liver damage and causing more accidents and injuries.

Prescribing for older adults is common. Some prescribed medicines such as benzodiazepines and opioids have a potential for abuse or dependence.

Mental health of the caregivers

Older adults with dementia and depression commonly receive support from spouses, other family members or friends. Caregivers commonly go through high levels of burden, stress, and depression. Providing psychosocial care to them should be included in the intervention packages for mental disorders of older adults.

Reading 出典: M. T. Yasamy, T. Dua M. Harper, S. Saxena, *Mental Health of Older Adults, Addressing a Growing Concern*, World Health Organization のウェブサイト〔WHO paper for the World Federation of Mental Health; http://www.who.int/mental_health/world-mental-health-day/WHO_paper_wmhd_2013.pdf（2015 年 1 月現在）〕より許可を得て転載.

9・2 Comprehension Questions

Based on the reading passage, circle T (true) or F (false) for each statement.

1. Approximately 20% of adults older than 55 in the world suffer from a mental disorder. (T , F)
2. Elder maltreatment is a risk factor to the health of older adults as well as an important human rights problem. (T , F)
3. According to the WHO and ADI, most people older than 60 years old are expected to suffer from dementia. (T , F)
4. The symptoms of depression in older adults are partly different from those in early life. (T , F)
5. We don't have to worry whether some prescribed medicines for treating mental disorders have the potential for abuse or dependence. (T , F)

9・3 Grammar

Choose the auxiliary verb from *will*, *can*, *could*, *should*, and *may* that best fits in each set of parentheses.

Target ➤ Auxiliary Verb

1. Depression ( ) be long-lasting or recurrent, substantially impairing an individual's ability to function at work or school or cope with daily life.
2. Dementia is the name for a group of symptoms caused by disorders that affect the brain. It is not a specific disease. People with dementia ( ) not be able to think well enough to do normal activities, such as getting dressed or eating.
3. At the first sign of a stroke, you ( ) get medical care right away. If blood vessels to your brain are blocked by blood clots, the doctor can give you a "clot-busting" drug.
4. AD is a major public health issue and will increasingly affect the health and well-being of the population. Unless the disease can be effectively treated or prevented, the number of Americans with AD ( ) increase significantly in the next two decades.
5. What if we could diagnose Alzheimer's before symptoms started? The hope is, future treatments ( ) then target the disease in its earliest stages, before irreversible brain damage or mental decline has occurred.

9・4 Medical Vocabulary

▶ 入院・検査・診断に関する用語と略語 (2)

Match each of the following abbreviated words with its meaning below and then translate the word into Japanese.

1. PET ( ) _____
2. CC ( ) _____
3. MRI ( ) _____
4. ADL ( ) _____
5. EEG ( ) _____
6. CT ( ) _____
7. US ( ) _____
8. ECG ( ) _____

a. magnetic resonance imaging
b. activities of daily living
c. chief complaint
d. electrocardiography
e. ultrasonography
f. positron-emission tomography
g. electroencephalogram
h. computed tomography

9・5　Writing
▶ **Giving advice (1)**

1. When do you feel stressed? When you feel stressed out, how can you get rid of your stress?

Hints !

I feel stressed when ....
I sleep and eat what I like.
I try to ....

_____
_____
_____
_____

2. When you see your friend or family member feeling terribly depressed, what sort of advice would you give him/her? Think about how you can help them and exchange your ideas with your group members.

_____
_____
_____
_____

COLUMN

高齢者の心のケアに目を向けよう！

　健康状態や生活機能は加齢によって低下し，環境の変化に適応する能力も減退してくる．したがって，高齢者においては，脳血管や骨の脆弱化，体温調節機能や内分泌機能の低下などに起因する体調不良に陥りやすい．もちろん，身体的な疾患に限らず，認知症やうつ病，不安症などの精神疾患に罹患する割合も上昇する．高齢者の精神疾患に対する治療の中心は，抗精神病薬による薬物療法であるが，薬物代謝能の低下から，有害作用を生じやすく，少量投与からの開始が基本となる．さらには，精神疾患は他の身体疾患と比較して，薬物療法が困難な場合もある．本章では，高齢者の精神疾患の現状，動向および治療に関して，世界的な視点から的確かつ簡潔にまとめられており，初学者でも，その概要を容易に把握できるように構成されている．将来，本分野における薬剤師としてのあり方について示唆を与える点でも興味深い内容となっている．

（徳山尚吾）

Chapter 10

Rheumatoid Arthritis

10・1 Reading

> 関節リウマチは，さまざまな症状をひき起こす可能性のある重病であるが，治療法の進歩により，関節の炎症の進行を緩和できるようになってきている。この章では，関節リウマチの定義，原因，疫学，診断法，治療法を学び，患者のQOLを維持するために医療従事者は何をすべきかを考えてみよう。

Track 10

What is rheumatoid arthritis?

Rheumatoid arthritis (commonly called RA) is a chronic disease that causes pain, stiffness, swelling and limited motion and function of many joints. While RA can affect any joints, the small joints in the hands and
5 feet tend to be involved most often. Inflammation sometimes can affect organs as well, for instance, the eyes or lungs.

rheumatoid arthritis 関節リウマチ（RA）

inflammation 炎症

What causes rheumatoid arthritis?

RA is an autoimmune disease. This means that certain cells of the immune system do not work properly and start attacking healthy
10 tissues—the joints in RA. The cause of RA is not known. Yet, new research is giving us a better idea of what makes the immune system attack the body and create inflammation. In RA, the focus of the inflammation is in the synovium. Immune cells release inflammation-causing chemicals. These chemicals can damage cartilage and bone.
15 Other things likely play a role in RA as well. For instance, genes that affect the immune system may make some people more prone to getting RA.

autoimmune 自己免疫(性)の

immune system 免疫系

synovium 滑膜

Who gets rheumatoid arthritis?

RA is the most common form of autoimmune arthritis, affecting more than 1.3 million Americans. Of these, about 75% are women. In fact, 1-3% of women may get RA in their lifetime. The disease most often begins between the fourth and sixth decades of life. However, RA can start at any age.

How is rheumatoid arthritis diagnosed?

RA can be hard to detect because it may begin with subtle symptoms, such as achy joints or a little stiffness in the morning. Also, many diseases behave like RA early on.

Diagnosis of RA depends on the symptoms and results of a physical exam, such as warmth, swelling and pain in the joints. Some blood tests also can help confirm RA.

X-rays can help in detecting RA, but may not show anything abnormal in early arthritis. Even so, these first X-rays may be useful later to show if the disease is progressing. Often, MRI and ultrasound scanning are done to help judge the severity of RA.

How is rheumatoid arthritis treated?

Therapy for RA has improved greatly in the past 30 years. Current treatments give most patients good or excellent relief of symptoms and let them keep functioning at, or near, normal levels. With the right medications, many patients can achieve "remission" —that is, have no signs of active disease.

Good control of RA requires early diagnosis and, at times, aggressive treatment. Thus, patients with a diagnosis of RA should begin their treatment with disease-modifying antirheumatic drugs—referred to as DMARDs. These drugs not only relieve symptoms but also slow progression of the disease. Often, doctors prescribe DMARDs along with nonsteroidal anti-inflammatory drugs (NSAIDs) and/or low-dose corticosteroids, to lower swelling, pain and fever. DMARDs have greatly improved the symptoms, function and quality of life for nearly all patients with RA.

Patients with more serious disease may need medications called "biologic agents." They can target the parts of the immune system and the signals that lead to inflammation and joint and tissue damage. These medications are also called DMARDs.

The best treatment of RA needs more than medicines alone. Patient education, such as how to cope with RA, also is important. Proper care requires the expertise of a team of providers, including rheumatologists, primary care physicians, pharmacists, and physical and occupational therapists.

Living with rheumatoid arthritis

Finding that you have a chronic illness is a life-changing event. It can cause worry and sometimes feelings of isolation or depression. Thanks to greatly improved treatments, these feelings tend to decrease with time as energy improves, and pain and stiffness decrease. Discuss these normal feelings with your health care providers. They can provide helpful information and resources.

出 典: *Reumatoid Arthritis*, American College of Rheumatology のウェブサイト〔http://www.rheumatology.org/practice/clinical/patients/diseases_and_conditions/ra.asp（2015年1月現在）〕より転載．© 2012 American College of Rheumatology.

10・2　Comprehension Questions

Based on the reading passage, circle T (true) or F (false) for each statement.

1. Rheumatoid arthritis, or RA for short, is triggered by a faulty immune system.　　　　　　　　　　　　　　　　　　　(T , F)
2. Women form a majority of the patients with RA in the U.S.　(T , F)
3. RA can be diagnosed more easily in its early stages.　(T , F)

4. Many patients with RA have not completely recovered from it so far.
(T , F)
5. Proper medication is the best possible way to treat RA. (T , F)

10・3 Grammar

In numbers 1, 2, 3, and 5, put appropriate word(s) starting with the letter presented in the parentheses. Refer to the Japanese at the end of the sentence to help you. In number 4, translate the underlined phrase into Japanese.

Target ▶ Adverb

COPD　Chronic obstructive pulmonary disease（慢性閉塞性肺疾患）

1. Keep ZUBSOLV® in a secure place away from children. If a child (a_____) takes ZUBSOLV®, this is a medical emergency and can result in death. Get emergency help right away. （もし子供が ZUBSOLV® を誤飲したら）
2. The more a person smokes, (t_____) that person will develop COPD. （ますますその人は COPD になるだろう）
3. (T_____), no tobacco products have met the requirements that would permit them to make claims of reduced risk or harm to users and nonusers of their regulated tobacco products. （今まで）
4. To further the FDA's understanding of the likely public health impact of the use of menthol in cigarettes, the FDA plans to support new research on the differences between menthol and nonmenthol cigarettes.
5. Although manufacturers have successfully made some medical devices less costly and (m_____) user-friendly, many devices are still too complex for a layperson to use safely and effectively without proper training. （コストを下げ，使いやすく）

10・4 Medical Vocabulary
▶ 入院・検査・診断に関する用語と略語（3）

Match each of the following abbreviated words with its meaning below and then translate the word into Japanese.

1. Adm   ( ) _____
2. I & O   ( ) _____
3. QOL   ( ) _____
4. OR   ( ) _____
5. Ps   ( ) _____
6. TPR   ( ) _____
7. ICU   ( ) _____
8. CPR   ( ) _____

a. quality of life
b. prescription

c. admission
   d. cardiopulmonary resuscitation
   e. temperature, pulse, respiration
   f. intake and output
   g. operation room
   h. intensive care unit

10・5 Writing
▶ **Giving advice (2)**

薬局を訪れた新しい患者さんに服薬指導と食事のアドバイスをします．以下の状況で，どのように対応しますか．会話をつくってみましょう．

George Brown was diagnosed with a lipid disorder. He has been taking 1 mg of LIVALO® daily for 20 days. He likes greasy food like French fries or ramen and eats them nearly every day late at night. He lives alone and mostly eats out.

Pharmacist: Hi, Mr. Brown, I understand that you are taking LIVALO®. _____

_____

_____

Mr. Brown: I like food like hamburgers and French fries, and eat ramen often late at night.

Pharmacist: Well, you might want to _____

_____

_____

COLUMN

関節リウマチ —— 痛みを和らげる治療から治癒する治療へ

関節リウマチ (RA) は，手や足の指をはじめとする多関節に炎症が起こり，関節の痛み，腫れ，破壊によって日常生活が困難になる病気です．1940 年代に RA の特効薬としてグルココルチコイドが登場するまで，アスピリンで"痛みを和らげる"しか治療法がない不治の病でした．画家 Pierre-Auguste Renoir も RA 患者として知られ，関節の痛みと変形に苦しみながらキャンバスと格闘したと伝えられています．1999 年，"関節破壊を食い止める"治療薬が登場しました．メトトレキサートです．これにより，RA 治療は劇的に変化しましたが，効果が不十分な症例もみられました．これを解決したのが，2003 年に登場したインフリキシマブ（炎症性サイトカインの一つである TNFα の働きを抑える抗体製剤）をはじめとする生物学的製剤です．生物学的製剤は，RA 治療の概念を革命的に変化させ，現在では，RA は"寛解する"あるいは"治癒する"病気になりつつあります．

（河野武幸）

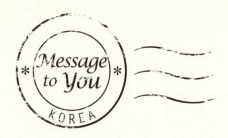

Pharmacy Education in Korea

Pharmacy education in Korea has a history of almost 100 years. What started in 1915 as a one-year program of modern pharmacy education, was changed to a two-year program in 1918, a three-year program in 1928, and a four-year program in 1945. Until that time, there was only one pharmacy school at Seoul National University. After that a second school of pharmacy for women was established at Ewha Woman's University in 1948. By 2008, there were a total of 20 colleges of pharmacy founded and they produced 1,200 graduates per year.

The goal of pharmacy education under the four-year education program was to produce both pharmacists and pharmacy scholars. In general, pharmacy schools followed a common curriculum with 12 mandatory subjects all of which are found on the Korean pharmacist licensure exam: Pharmacology, Biochemistry, Hygienic Chemistry, Microbiology, Pharmaceutical Qualitative Analysis, Pharmaceutical Quantitative Analysis, Pharmaceutics, Pharmacognosy, Inorganic Pharmaceutical Chemistry, Organic Pharmaceutical Chemistry, Korean Pharmacopoeia, and Acts on Pharmaceutical Affairs & Control of Narcotics. Besides these core subjects, each pharmacy school manages elective subjects according to their specific education goals to nurture competent pharmacy experts. They include: Medicinal Chemistry, Biotechnology, Clinical Pharmacy, Pharmacy Management, Industrial Pharmacy, etc....

In 2009, Korea made a turning point and the pharmacy education system changed to a six-year program. In the same year, additional new pharmacy schools were founded at 15 different universities, and consequently the number of pharmacy graduates is expected to be 1,600 per year from 2015. Under the six-year education system, pharmacy applicants should complete pre-pharmacy prerequisite coursework in a 2-year time period and achieve good marks on the Pharmacy Education Eligibility Test. In this regard, the new system is sometimes referred to as a 2+4 pharmacy education system.

Under the former four-year pharmacy program, the graduates were often confronted with a considerable gap between the subjects they had studied in the pharmaceutical sciences and actual pharmacy practice in clinical settings. Therefore, there a need and call for pharmacy practice training. The global development of biopharmacy also led to a call for a new curriculum in pharmacy education. As a result, several significant changes took place in the new pharmacy education system, the two largest of which were the extension of clinical pharmacy and the integration of 1,400 hours of practical training. In addition, modules covering biopharmacy and social pharmacy have also been introduced.

The new pharmacy education has stressed the importance of clinical pharmacy that emphasizes Pharmacotherapy and other subjects for patient-centered services such as pharmaceutical care and communication skills. The practical training consists of 800 hours of mandatory practice and 600 hours of advanced practice. During the mandatory practice hours, students must perform more than 10 weeks of hospital pharmacy practice and five weeks of community pharmacy practice. During the advanced practice hours, students have a chance to get advanced work experience within a single site according to their future job prospects. For advanced practice training, students make a choice of one practice place inform the following: community pharmacy, hospital pharmacy, pharmaceutical industry, research laboratories, or health-related government administrative office.

As the education system has changed and pharmacy students have more chances of experiencing and understanding actual work of several different fields, I, in the aspect of a pharmacy educator, expect that graduates will expand their future careers to other less well-known areas than community and hospital pharmacists, while most of the former four-year pharmacy graduates currently work as a pharmacist in community and hospital pharmacy settings.

Japan has already changed their pharmacy education into a six-year program that comes from a government-driven initiative, which is different from that here in Korea. Although the course of change and final frame of pharmacy education is different between our two countries, the goal of pharmacy education is the same to foster pharmacists and pharmacy scholars who will devote their life to counselling patients on the proper use of medications and to the advancement of the health and pharmaceutical sciences. I hope you do your best in your pharmacy studies and best of luck with your future careers.

> Jung-Ae Kim, Ph.D.
> Professor, College of Pharmacy, Yeungnam University

Chapter 11
Dabigatran Versus Warfarin in Patients With Mechanical Heart Valves

11・1 Reading

dabigatran ダビガトラン．直接トロンビン阻害薬（商品名プラザキサ®）〈効能効果は，非弁膜症性心房細動患者における虚血性脳卒中および全身性塞栓症の発症抑制〉

この章で扱う疾病は発生頻度が高く，現場の薬剤師がその薬物療法に関して専門性の高い問い合わせなどに遭遇する可能性がある．以下の内容は，病院薬剤部の薬剤師が医師から受けた，直接トロンビン阻害薬の使用上の注意に関する問い合わせと，一次資料の文献から科学的根拠に基づく情報を収集し適切に対応した実例を基にしている．

事例：あなたが，薬剤師として働いている，ある大学医学部附属病院の薬剤部医薬品情報室に，"人工弁置換術後の患者に対してプラザキサ®（直接トロンビン阻害薬，ダビガトラン）が使用禁忌となっている理由"について，医師より問い合わせがあった．その根拠となる論文を "dabigatran" および "mechanical heart valve" から検索エンジンで探したところ，以下の論文がヒットした．J. W. Eikelboom, et al., "Dabigatran Versus Warfarin in Patients With Mechanical Heart Valves", *The New England Journal of Medicine*, 369（13），1206～1214（2013）．

et al. およびその他の人々〈ラテン語 et alii の略〉

（注：この論文の内容を評価するために必要な臨床データが書かれている部分を以下に抜粋した．実際の業務では情報を集めるべき箇所を自身で選定する．研究デザイン，臨床試験参加者の選定と割付，症例数の設定，評価項目，結果の提示とデータ解析，臨床的な有意さと外的妥当性などに注意しながら，論文の根拠の質を精査するのが一般的である．）

oral direct thrombin inhibitor 経口直接トロンビン阻害薬

warfarin ワルファリン，抗凝固薬〈効能効果は，血栓塞栓症（静脈血栓症，心筋梗塞症，肺塞栓症，脳塞栓症，緩徐に進行する脳血栓症など）の治療および予防〉

atrial fibrillation 心房細動

mechanical heart valves 人工心臓弁

aortic- or mitral-valve replacement 大動脈または僧帽弁置換

Abstract

Background

Dabigatran is an oral direct thrombin inhibitor that has been shown to be an effective alternative to warfarin in patients with atrial fibrillation. We evaluated the use of dabigatran in patients with mechanical heart valves.

Methods

In this phase 2 dose-validation study, we studied two populations of patients: those who had undergone aortic- or mitral-valve replacement within the past 7 days and those who had undergone such replacement at least 3 months earlier. Patients were randomly assigned in a 2:1 ratio to receive either dabigatran or warfarin. The selection of the initial dabigatran dose (150, 220, or 300 mg twice daily) was based on kidney function. Doses were adjusted to obtain a trough plasma level of at least 50 ng per milliliter. The warfarin dose was adjusted to obtain an international normalized ratio of 2 to 3 or 2.5 to 3.5 on the basis of thromboembolic risk. The primary end point was the trough plasma level of dabigatran.

Results

The trial was terminated prematurely after the enrollment of 252 patients because of an excess of thromboembolic and bleeding events among patients in the dabigatran group. In the as-treated analysis, dose adjustment or discontinuation of dabigatran was required in 52 of 162 patients (32%). Ischemic or unspecified stroke occurred in 9 patients (5%) in the dabigatran group and in no patients in the warfarin group; major bleeding occurred in 7 patients (4%) and 2 patients (2%), respectively. All patients with major bleeding had pericardial bleeding.

Conclusions

The use of dabigatran in patients with mechanical heart valves was associated with increased rates of thromboembolic and bleeding complications, as compared with warfarin, thus showing no benefit and an excess risk....

Methods

Study design and oversight

RE-ALIGN was a prospective, randomized, phase 2, open-label trial with blinded end-point adjudication. The trial was conducted at 39 centers in 10 countries.... The trial protocol was approved by the ethics committee at each participating site.... The data were collected and analyzed by Boehringer Ingelheim, U.K....

Patients and randomization

...Patients were eligible for inclusion if they were between the ages of 18 and 75 years and were undergoing implantation of a mechanical bileaflet valve in the aortic or mitral position or both (population A) or if they had undergone implantation of a mechanical bileaflet mitral valve (with or without mechanical bileaflet aortic-valve replacement) more than 3 months before randomization (population B).... All patients provided written informed consent before enrollment. Patients were randomly assigned to receive dabigatran or warfarin in a ratio of 2:1....

Results

Clinical outcome

...A major bleeding episode occurred in 7 patients (4%) in the dabigatran group and 2 patients (2%) in the warfarin group, and bleeding of any type occurred in 45 patients (27%) and 10 patients (12%), respectively (hazard ratio, 2.45; 95% CI, 1.23 to 4.86; P=0.01).... A consistent pattern of increased bleeding events in the dabigatran group was evident in both population A and population B. However, all major bleeding occurred in patients who underwent randomization within 1 week after cardiac surgery (population A). All patients with major bleeding had pericardial bleeding, which occurred within 2 weeks after surgery in 5 patients in the dabigatran group and 2 patients in the warfarin group....

Discussion

The primary goal of RE-ALIGN was to validate a new dabigatran dosing regimen for the prevention of thromboembolic complications in patients with mechanical heart valves. However, the trial was stopped early because of an excess of thromboembolic and bleeding events in the dabigatran group, as compared with the warfarin group. Most thromboembolic events among patients in the dabigatran group occurred in population A (patients who had started a study drug within 7 days after valve surgery), with fewer occurring in population B (patients who had undergone valve implantation more than 3 months before randomization). Excess bleeding events among patients receiving dabigatran occurred in the two study populations....

出 典：J. W. Eikelboom, et al., "Dabigatran Versus Warfarin in Patients With Mechanical Heart Valves", *The New England Journal of Medicine*, 369(13), 1206～1214(2013) より許可を得て転載．Copyright ©2013 Massachusetts Medical Society. All rights reserved.

11・2 Comprehension Questions

医療従事者からの問い合わせに回答するための情報について，以下の問いに答えてください．

1. この研究の"主要目的（primary goal）"は何ですか．日本語で答えなさい．
   例：<u>何かの処置を受けた患者</u>を対象に，<u>使用した何かの薬</u>を投与した後の健康被害を予防できるかを検討した臨床試験である．（<u>下線部分</u>を実際の用語で置き換える．）
2. 研究方法（デザイン）は，前向き（prospective）の介入研究（randomized trial）です．"介入群（研究の対象者）"が服用した薬は何ですか．また，"非介入群（介入群と対照される人たち）"は何をするよう伝えられましたか．次の中から選びなさい．
   ①何もしない　　②プラセボを飲む　③他の薬剤を飲む
3. 臨床試験は10カ国39施設で行われましたが，参加者は何人まで登録（enrollment）されましたか．年齢は何歳から何歳まででしたか．どのような患者が対象（eligible）となりましたか．（ヒント：研究集団AとBが選択された．）
4. 臨床試験は，途中で中断（terminated prematurely）しなければなりませんでしたが，その理由を簡潔に書きなさい．また，その判断をした根拠となる具体的な数字あるいは百分率は何ですか．
5. 研究はどう結論付けられましたか．あなたが問い合わせを受けた薬剤師だったとして，医師にはどのように回答すべきですか．

11・3 Grammar

Put a preposition, *at*, *by*, *in*, *to*, or *with* in each set of parentheses to make each sentence meaningful.

Target ▶ Preposition

1. The FDA is investigating reports that carbendazim, a fungicide, is present (　　) low levels in some orange juice products.
2. Diabetes-associated chronic kidney disease (CKD) continues to be a major contributor (　　) morbidity and mortality in the U.S. and the world.
3. The most cost-effective strategy for preventing rabies in people is (　　) eliminating rabies in dogs through vaccination.
4. Mental health is a state of well-being (　　) which an individual realizes his or her own abilities, can cope with the normal stresses of life, can work productively and is able to make a contribution to his or her community.
5. (　　) the exception of color additives, a manufacturer may use any ingredient in the formulation of a cosmetic that does not cause the cosmetic to be adulterated or misbranded under the FD&C Act.

FD&C Act　the Federal Food, Drug, and Cosmetic Act

11・4　Medical Vocabulary
▶ 検査値の用語と略語 (1)

Match each of the following abbreviated words with its meaning below and then translate the word into Japanese.

1. TP 　(　)　_____
2. Alb 　(　)　_____
3. UA 　(　)　_____
4. BUN 　(　)　_____
5. Cr 　(　)　_____
6. eGFR 　(　)　_____
7. ALT 　(　)　_____
8. AST 　(　)　_____

a. uric acid
b. estimated glomerular filtration rate
c. serum total protein
d. aspartate aminotransferase
e. alanine aminotransferase
f. serum albumin
g. blood urea nitrogen
h. serum creatinine

11・5　Writing
▶ **Sharing information (1)**

興味ある病気の治療薬と出ているジェネリック薬品の特徴を調べ，英語で発表してみましょう．

Hints !

... is a drug for....

... is a generic medication of....

___

COLUMN

経口抗凝固薬ダビガトランに対する期待とリスク

　ダビガトランはワルファリン以来，約50年ぶり（2011年）に発売された経口の抗凝固薬（トロンビン阻害薬）です．心房細動などで血流のうっ滞した心臓内に生じた血栓が，脳血管に詰まる脳塞栓症の発症予防が適応です．ワルファリンは，定期的な血液検査で用量を調整する必要があり，納豆などの食事制限もあり，生涯にわたり服用する場合もある薬剤としては制限の多いものです．ダビガトランはこうした血液検査，用量調整や食事制限などを必要としない，臨床的に使いやすい薬として期待されました．抗凝固薬の最も注意すべき有害反応は出血ですが，出血性合併症はワルファリンよりも少ないと報告されていました（RE-LY試験，2009年）．しかし，日本での発売直後から，期待に反し，消化管出血などの出血による死亡例が多数報告される事態となり，本剤の添付文書に出血リスクに関する"警告"が加えられました．ダビガトランは出血リスクをモニターできず，解毒薬もないため，現在は慎重な投与が求められています．　　　（木内祐二）

Licensed to Work as a Pharmacist in Both Japan and America

Dear Japanese student pharmacists,

Hello, my name is Kanako Rosario (Miyairi). I graduated from Keio University Faculty of Pharmacy (back when the school was called Kyoritsu College of Pharmacy). After graduating, I went to Nova Southeastern University College of Pharmacy in the United States, and earned a Doctor of Pharmacy (Pharm.D.) Degree.

I am currently a pharmacist at a community/retail pharmacy in Florida. I find it very rewarding that community pharmacy is the last stop before patients receive their medications, and we play a pivotal role in assuring patients' medication efficacy and safety. Before I get more into detail with why I feel working in community pharmacies is worthwhile, I would like to briefly touch on why I chose this path.

One of the many reasons why I love being a pharmacist in the US is that there are many career paths available to us. From clinical sites to research to academia, which a lot of times combines both aspects of clinical practice and research, we have a great variety of career paths to choose from, and with your effort and a bit of luck, you can go into any path at any given time of your career. Upon graduating, I was facing the time to make a decision as to which path I was going to take. I wanted to work in a clinical field, so my choices were either community pharmacy or hospital. In the US, the last year of pharmacy school is all rotations, so from my rotation experience, I thought to myself, "If I wanted more direct patient interaction as part of my daily practice, community is the way to go, but if I wanted more interaction with fellow healthcare workers, I would want to go into a hospital setting." Thus, I had made my decision. I wanted more direct patient interaction, so I chose the community pharmacy path.

As of today, I have made a decision to try out the clinical route in a community setting. So far I have found this to be challenging, yet rewarding. Since the vast majority of your communication is going to be with your patients that come to your pharmacy, the very unique thing about this setting is that you need to be ready and know how to explain things in layman's terms. For example, if a patient is complaining of an upset stomach, and they want to know if they should take Famotidine or Omeprazole, you will confuse the patient if your tell him/her, " Try the Famotidine first since that is an H2-blocker, not a PPI." Instead, I would tell the patient (of course do not forget to ask him/her if they have tried any of the stomach remedies and have had success or allergic reactions first), "Try the Famotidine first since you might not need a drug that strong as Omeprazole. It might take some time before you feel the relief, but try it out for a couple of days. Make sure you don't take it too long before consulting your doctor."

I also like the fact that patients who come to your pharmacy are many times regular patients. In other words, you will see them every month or every three months. You will get to know them, they will get to know you, so I feel closer to them and more involved in their personal healthcare needs. If they feel comfortable talking to you, it is much more likely that they will share critical health information with you, and I feel that is something that's only possible in a good community pharmacy setting. They will ask you all sorts of questions that you would never imagine, so be ready for the fun and challenge on a daily basis.

Practicing in the US, there will always be an opportunity that fits your personality as a pharmacist. In the future, although I am practicing as a community pharmacist now, I might try out a hospital route, I might even consider research one day. As a closing statement, I just wanted to share with you young students that as long as you have the drive and passion, it might take time and much hard work, but I am hopeful that you will find a great career that you like.

Good luck to you all!

Sincerely,

Kanako Rosario (Miyairi)

Chapter 12
More Drugs Show Promise in Fighting Hepatitis C

12・1 Reading

> ウイルス感染で生じるC型肝炎．従来の抗ウイルス薬には重い副作用という問題があるので，治療の質を高めるために新薬の開発が続いている．本章ではそうした新薬の臨床試験について報じるニュース記事を読む．記事のもととなった論文 "Faldaprevir and Deleobuvir for HCV Genotype 1 Infection" を *New England Journal of Medicine* のウェブサイトで閲覧すると，さらに理解が深まるだろう．

standard therapy 標準的治療〈科学的根拠に基づいて，現時点で最善とされる治療法〉

An experimental drug duo may cure some cases of the liver disease hepatitis C, without the severe side effects of standard therapy, a new clinical trial suggests.

The study, of 362 people with chronic hepatitis C, found that the new drugs—combined with one older drug—cleared the virus from up to 69 percent of patients. And that was without having to use interferon, a difficult-to-take injection drug that is part of the current therapy.

Experts said the findings, published in the Aug. 15 issue of the *New England Journal of Medicine*, are another step forward in vastly improving hepatitis C treatment.

U.S. Food and Drug Administration (FDA) 米国食品医薬品局

Dozens of drugs are in development, and some are currently being considered for approval by the U.S. Food and Drug Administration (FDA).

"These are very exciting times in hepatitis C treatment," said Dr. Michael Saag, an infectious disease specialist at the University of Alabama at Birmingham who was not involved in the new study.

Hepatitis C is a liver infection usually passed through contact with infected blood. For most people, the infection becomes chronic, which can eventually lead to scarring of the liver (cirrhosis) or liver cancer years later.

That happens only in a minority of people. "But we have no way of knowing in advance who will develop cirrhosis or cancer," Saag said.

The current drug regimen for chronic hepatitis C includes interferon, plus an older oral drug called ribavirin, and either one of two drugs just approved in the last couple of years, called telaprevir and boceprevir. That combo cures about 68 percent to 75 percent of people with the most common strain of hepatitis C, called genotype 1.

The problem is, treatment lasts for months and almost always causes substantial side effects.

Interferon is especially hard to take, with side effects ranging from sleep problems and mood swings, to nausea and diarrhea, to muscle pain, fever and fatigue.

"There is a great desire to be able to cure hepatitis C without interferon," said Saag, who also serves on the Infectious Diseases Society of America's hepatitis task force.

In the new study, funded by drugmaker Boehringer Ingelheim, German researchers tested two experimental drugs called faldaprevir and deleobuvir against hepatitis C genotype 1.

The investigators randomly assigned 362 patients to one of five groups. Each group received the two new drugs. Four groups also took ribavirin, while the fifth did not.

In the end, the ribavirin proved necessary, Saag pointed out. Three months after their treatment ended, anywhere from 52 percent to 69 percent of patients on all three drugs were hepatitis free, depending on the dose and how long they took the medications.

In contrast, only 39 percent of patients who did not take ribavirin were free of the virus.

The benefits also depended on which virus subtype patients had. Of those with genotype 1b, up to 85 percent were hepatitis free three months after treatment. That compared with no better than 47 percent of patients with type 1a.

There are still questions, and later-stage trials of the new drugs are continuing, said study leader Dr. Stefan Zeuzem, of Goethe University Medical Center, in Frankfurt.

As for side effects, nearly all of the study patients had some, including rash, nausea, vomiting and diarrhea. But for most, those problems were mild, Zeuzem's team noted.

"Interferon side effects are certainly worse than side effects observed with faldaprevir and deleobuvir," Zeuzem said.

"It looks like severe side effects were not common," Saag agreed. But, he said, "the main problem with these drugs is that you still have to use ribavirin."

Ribavirin is more tolerable than interferon, but it destroys red blood cells and can cause serious fatigue and other problems.

出 典：A. Norton, *More Drugs Show Promise in Fighting Hepatitis C*, HealthDay のウェブサイト〔Aug 14, 2013（HealthDay News）http://consumer.healthday.com/cancer-information 5/mis-cancer-news-102/expcrimental-drugs-may-cure-some-hepatitis-c-cases-679239.html（2015 年 1 月現在）〕より許可を得て転載．Copyright ©2013 HealthDay. All rights reserved.

12・2 Comprehension Questions

Select the best answer for each question.

1. Why is it necessary to develop new treatments for hepatitis C?
    a. Because the number of patients with hepatitis C is increasing.
    b. Because current treatments are no longer effective.
    c. Because drug-resistant strains of the hepatitis C virus have emerged.
    d. Because current treatments cause severe side effects.
2. What was discovered in the clinical trial?
    a. The combination of faldaprevir, deleobuvir and ribavirin is effective in eliminating the hepatitis C virus.

b. The combination of faldaprevir and deleobuvir never causes severe side effects.
c. Interferon is necessary to treat hepatitis C.
d. Faldaprevir and deleobuvir are more effective against hepatitis C genotype 1a than against genotype 1b.
3. Which is true of Dr. Saag?
   a. He works for the FDA.
   b. He conducted a new study.
   c. He specializes in infectious diseases.
   d. He is completely positive about the usefulness of the new therapy.
4. How many participants experienced side effects?
   a. All of them.
   b. Most of them.
   c. A few of them.
   d. Almost none of them.

12・3 Grammar

Choose the best word from *given*, *if*, *provided*, *that*, *where*, and *whether* to put into each set of parentheses.

Target ➤ Conjunction and Relative

1. However, people living with dementia can still have a good quality of life throughout the dementia journey, (   ) the right long-term care plan is in place and being delivered.
2. It is often claimed that people with dementia would prefer to live at home for as long as possible cared for by their family, that this option is associated with better quality of life, and (   ) care at home is cheaper than care in a care home.
3. Vector-borne diseases are commonly found in tropical and sub-tropical regions and places (   ) access to safe drinking-water and sanitation systems is problematic.

   vector-borne 生物(動物)媒介の

4. We will use the mouse as a model system to study (   ) flavor additives increase nicotine levels, lead to alterations in breathing, and (   ) they cause lung inflammation and exaggeration of asthma.
5. (   ) the lack of agreed global standards for ABR surveillance, the reported proportions of resistance should be interpreted with caution.

   ABR antibacterial resistance (抗菌薬耐性)

12・4 Medical Vocabulary

▶ 検査値の用語と略語 (2)

Match each of the following abbreviated words with its meaning below and then translate the word into Japanese.

1. γ-GTP   ( ) _____
2. LDH   ( ) _____
3. ALP   ( ) _____

4. PRA (　) _____
5. CK　 (　) _____
6. ChE (　) _____
7. TC　 (　) _____
8. LDL-C (　) _____
9. HDL-C (　) _____

a. alkaline phosphatase
b. cholinesterase
c. creatine kinase
d. lactase dehydrogenase
e. plasma renin activity
f. high-density lipoprotein cholesterol
g. γ-glutamyl transpeptidase
h. total cholesterol
i. low-density lipoprotein cholesterol

12・5　Writing
▶ **Sharing information (2)**

1. 薬の副作用に関する表現について英訳しましょう．
　(1) この薬には以下のような副作用が起こりえます．

　_____

　_____

　_____

　_____

　　口の乾き　_____

　　だるさ　　_____

　　湿疹　　　_____

　(2) もしこのような症状が起こったら，この薬の服用をやめて薬剤師や医師に相談ください．

　_____

　_____

　_____

　_____

2. 起こりうる薬の副作用について調べ英語で表現しなさい．

　　When taking (　　　　　), (　　　　　　　　　　　　　)
may occur.

COLUMN

新時代を迎えた C 型慢性肝炎の治療

　C 型肝炎ウイルス（HCV）の血液を介した感染により発症する C 型急性肝炎は，高率に（約 70～80％）慢性化します．C 型慢性肝炎は，時間をかけて肝硬変から肝細胞がんへと進展し，日本では肝硬変と肝細胞がんの約 70％は HCV 陽性といわれます．このことから，C 型肝炎患者からの HCV の早期排除が，肝硬変と肝細胞がんを予防し，生命予後を改善するために最も重要な治療戦略となっています．C 型慢性肝炎の治療はインターフェロン（IFN）製剤が中心でしたが，抗ウイルス薬（RNA 依存性 RNA ポリメラーゼ阻害薬）のリバビリンが 2001 年に認可され，さらに，ポリエチレングリコール（PEG）と結合し，週 1 回の注射で持続するようにした PEG-IFN も開発され，治療効果が向上しました．しかし，HCV のウイルス量や遺伝子型によって IFN やリバビリンによる効果が異なることも明らかになりました．有効性を上げるために，プロテアーゼ阻害薬のシメプレビル，テラプレビル，アスナプレビル，NS5A 阻害薬ダクラタスビルなどの新機序の薬剤が続々と開発，認可され，C 型慢性肝炎の治療は新時代を迎えようとしています．　　　（木内祐二）

Chapter 13

End of the Road: Diabetes Care When Insulin May Not Be an Option

13・1 Reading

> 糖尿病には標準的な治療方法はあるものの，生活習慣や社会環境，薬など，さまざまな方面から患者一人一人に合わせて治療方針が設定される．そのため内容が複雑化し，治療が困難になるケースが問題となっている．このようななか，米国では糖尿病専門の薬剤師が活躍し，患者の糖尿病治療に大きな役割を果たしている．

commercial driver's license（CDL） 商業用車両運転免許（証）

metformin メトホルミン〈ビグアナイド系経口糖尿病治療薬．肝臓で糖の合成を抑える〉

glipizide グリピジド〈スルホニル尿素系経口糖尿病治療薬．インスリン分泌を促進する〉

A1C HbA1C（ヘモグロビン A1C）〈赤血球中の酸素を運ぶヘモグロビンに血液中の糖が結合したもの．過去1〜2カ月間の平均血糖値を表す〉

clinical inertia 治療効果が停滞する状態

Department of Transportation（DOT）physical 米国交通局の行う免許取得に関わる身体検査

hyperglycemia 高血糖

polyphagia 過食

polydipsia 多飲

polyuria 多尿

self-monitoring of blood glucose（SMBG） 血糖自己測定

J.U. is a 53-year-old man with uncomplicated Type 2 diabetes who requires a commercial driver's license (CDL) for his occupation as a truck driver and mechanic. His diabetes was controlled with increasing doses of metformin and glipizide during the first 4 years after his diagnosis. Despite nutrition counseling, diabetes education classes, and physician visits every 3-6 months, nonadherence with therapeutic lifestyle changes contributed to his A1C fluctuating between 7.2 and 10.2% over 3 years. His health care provider recommended insulin therapy numerous times, but J.U.'s needle fear, lifestyle preferences, and fear of losing his job led to patient refusal and clinical inertia.

He is seen for an urgent appointment after his Department of Transportation (DOT) physical was failed for hyperglycemia (glucose >200 mg/dl) and significant levels of glucose in the urine. He reports fatigue, polyphagia, polydipsia, and polyuria. He has not been compliant with self-monitoring of blood glucose (SMBG) or recommended therapeutic lifestyle changes.

At the time of this visit, his diabetes medication regimen consists of metformin 1,000 mg twice daily and glipizide 10 mg twice daily with meals. His A1C is 8.1%, weight is 207 lb (BMI 32.5 kg/m^2), blood pressure is 110/72 mmHg, pulse is 80 bpm, serum creatinine is 0.9 mg/dl, total cholesterol is 116 mg/dl, triglyceride level is 207 mg/dl, LDL cholesterol is 46 mg/dl, and HDL cholesterol is 29 mg/dl.

He has a known history of hyperlipidemia treated with a statin, hypertension treated with an ACE inhibitor, and gastroesophageal reflux disease treated with a proton pump inhibitor. He has smoked two packs of cigarettes per day for 32 years, with multiple failed quit attempts, and denies alcohol or illicit drug use.

J.U. provides the primary source of income for his family and has financial difficulties. Having to stop work, even for a brief period, would be financially devastating to his family. His physician signs a medical examination form certifying that his diabetes will be closely monitored and managed, which will allow the patient 6 months to control his diabetes and pass the DOT physical. The patient is referred to the clinical pharmacist to provide diabetes disease state management as part of a collaborative practice agreement within a patient-centered medical home.

Progress after pharmacist referral

During frequent visits, the pharmacist reinforces diabetes education, including lifestyle modifications, diabetes symptoms, complications, goals of care, SMBG, and medications. Each session concludes with patient goal-setting.

Diabetes testing supplies are obtained through the patient's insurance with low out-of-pocket costs. The pharmacist switches his glipizide prescription to the extended-release formulation to optimize therapy and initiates sitagliptin 100 mg daily. Manufacturer rebates allow J.U. to obtain sitagliptin at a low cost.

fasting blood glucose level　空腹時血糖値

pioglitazone　ピオグリタゾン〈チアゾリジン系経口糖尿病治療薬．筋肉や肝臓でのインスリンの働きを高める作用〉

quadruple　4種の

In a period of 8 weeks, J.U.'s average fasting blood glucose level improves to 154 mg/dl, and his A1C improves to 7.9%. A shared decision is made among the patient, his provider, and the pharmacist to initiate pioglitazone 15 mg daily. After 3 months of quadruple oral therapy, his A1C is 6.8%, and weight gain has been limited to 3.5 lb with strict diet and exercise.

When insulin is not an option, it is not the end of the road. Personalized, intensive, and frequent disease state management of diabetes is an effective strategy. Many noninsulin treatment options exist and can be combined to achieve blood glucose targets.

The burden of diabetes is often overwhelming. Social, cultural, and financial issues often become barriers to optimal care. Regulatory restrictions add another level of complexity to the adequate treatment of patients with diabetes. Clinicians need to be aware of federal and state regulations regarding their patients' occupation and disease state before making treatment decisions. Alternative employment opportunities are not always an option, and taking time from work to obtain necessary exemptions may prove costly to such patients. Relying on other members of the health care team, including pharmacists, diabetes educators, and dietitians, can help with the complexity of treating and educating patients with diabetes.

出　典：P. M. Stranges, J. M. Tingen "End of the Road: Diabetes Care When Insulin May Not Be an Option", *Clinical Diabetes*, 32(2), 87〜89（2014）より許可を得て転載．Copyright ©2014 American Diabetes Association.

13・2　Comprehension Questions

Answer the following questions in English.

1. What type of license is required to work as a truck driver?

　

2. Why did J. U. refuse insulin therapy?

3. What therapy options exist for patients with Type 2 diabetes when insulin therapy is refused or not plausible?

_____

4. After the referral, what did the pharmacist do to achieve the therapeutic target?

_____

5. Why should physicians rely on other members of the health care team to assist in treating patients with diabetes?

_____

13・3 Grammar

Rewrite each underlined part of the following sentences into ones with conjunctions, if necessary, and verbs.

Target ▶ Participle

1. <u>Once considered a high-income country problem</u>, overweight and obesity are now on the rise in low- and middle-income countries, particularly in urban settings.
2. During an asthma attack, the lining of the bronchial tubes swells, <u>causing</u> the airways to narrow and reducing the flow of air into and out of the lungs.
3. The muscles gradually become paralyzed, <u>starting</u> at the site of the bite or scratch.
4. When water comes from improved and more accessible sources, people spend less time and effort in physically collecting it, <u>meaning</u> they can be productive in other ways.
5. For years, scientists <u>trying</u> to develop a malaria vaccine have been stymied by the malaria parasite's ability to transform itself and "hide" in the liver and red blood cells of an infected person to avoid detection by the immune system.

stymie　妨害する

13・4 Medical Vocabulary

▶ 検査値の用語と略語（3）

Match each of the following abbreviated words with its meaning below and then translate the word into Japanese.

1. TG　　（　）_____
2. AMY　（　）_____
3. GA　　（　）_____
4. GTT　 （　）_____
5. WBC　（　）_____
6. RBC　（　）_____

7. Plt ( ) _____
8. HB ( ) _____
9. Hct ( ) _____

a. platelet count
b. glucose tolerance test
c. white blood cell count
d. triglyceride
e. hematocrit
f. red blood cell count
g. glycated albumin
h. amylase
i. glycated hemoglobin

13・5 Writing
▶ Giving advice (3)

1. Advise your patient who finds it difficult to take medicine regularly.

   Mr. Wilson, if it is difficult to take medicine regularly, you should
   _____
   _____
   _____
   _____

2. Advise your patient with mild influenza.

   Ms. Foxley, make sure to drink fluids from time to time and
   _____
   _____
   _____
   _____

COLUMN

DPP-4 阻害薬

新しい糖尿病治療薬である DPP-4 阻害薬は, 日本で 2009 年以降に発売されましたが, 2 型糖尿病の治療を大きく変える可能性があります. その効果は, 血糖降下作用を示すインクレチンを分解する酵素を阻害して, インスリンの分泌を促進しグルカゴンの分泌を抑制することなどに基づきます. インクレチンは食事による糖吸収が刺激になって分泌されますので, DPP-4 阻害薬は血糖値に応じた血糖降下作用を示すのが特徴です. したがって, スルホニル尿素薬にみられるような低血糖発作のリスクは少なく, 患者 QOL の面からも優れています. また, DPP-4 阻害薬は, ビグアナイド系薬のように乳酸アシドーシスのリスクはほとんどなく, 糖尿病性腎症でも安全に投与できるものもあります. さらに DPP-4 阻害薬は, 肥満になりにくいとともに, 欧米人に比べて BMI が小さい日本人の糖尿病患者に対してより効果的であることがわかっています. まだ歴史の浅い薬ですが, DPP-4 阻害薬には大きな期待が寄せられています. (賀川義之)

Evolution of Pharmacy Education in Taiwan

Pharmacy education in Taiwan began in the 1950s, starting with a four-year B.S.Pharm. program. After a period of chaos from 1966 to 1999, pharmacy education unified as a four- to five-year B.S.Pharm. program from the year 2000. These programs have to cover drug research and development, community pharmacy, hospital pharmacy, and the drug industry. Each year around 1,000 pharmacy students graduate from seven universities. Only 50% of pharmacy students will pass the licensure examination each year, but this still allows us to get about 1,000 new pharmacists per year. Around 70% of pharmacists are registered. Among them, 22%, 31%, and 26%, respectively, work at hospitals, community pharmacies, and private clinics. The remaining 20% work in drug companies, mostly for marketing, sales, clinical trials, and registration.

All the pharmacy students in Taiwan have to fulfill practice-experience hours before graduation. Because of the advancement in hospital pharmacy practice since the 1990s (e.g., drug information and analysis services, drug use evaluation, drug protocol management, drug therapy monitoring, therapeutic drug monitoring and pharmacokinetic services, adverse drug reaction monitoring and reporting, medical round participation, medication reconciliation, patient counseling and education, pharmacy-managed clinics, and information technology application in medication management and use), and the lack of prescriptions in community pharmacies, a standardized 640-hour practice experience in an accredited teaching hospital was emphasized since 2005, and has been required for sitting the licensure examination since 2013. In recent years, community pharmacists try to devote themselves to long-term care, home care and health promotion. We hope that community pharmacy practice will be part of the licensure requirement in the future.

A two-year clinical pharmacy or hospital pharmacy master's program with patient-oriented courses and 36-week advanced clinical experiential training was developed in 1993 at National Cheng-Kung University and National Taiwan University to foster pharmacy professionals devoted to the clinical services, teaching and research, and to advance the quality of pharmacotherapy and clinical research in Taiwan. A similar program has been developed in the other three universities with diverse content. However, only 20 to 30 students nationwide may be admitted each year.

In 2009, National Taiwan University pioneered the first six-year Pharm.D. program in Taiwan. After five years of a parallel four-year B.S. Pharm and six-year Pharm.D.

program, beginning in 2014, the school will only offer the six-year Pharm.D. program. This program follows the Accreditation Council of Pharmacy Education (ACPE) standards and provides integrated courses to excel in pharmacy education. In addition to hospital and community pharmacy externship, students must finish 36-week advance pharmacy practice experiences (APPE). The APPE consists of 24 weeks of core courses in hospital settings and 12 weeks of elective courses in a community pharmacy setting. Students can choose pharmacy administration, industrial pharmacy, pharmaceutical manufacturer, research, hospital pharmacy, or community pharmacy as electives according to their interest. There are also industrial pharmacy and pharmaceutical manufacturer externships as elective courses.

From the year of 2014, three out of the eight pharmacy schools in Taiwan offer a Pharm.D. program for about 110 students per year, which will account for 11% of pharmacy students. These programs are expected to equip pharmacists with strong therapeutic, clinical, and administrative competency to meet the needs of the health-care system, health-care administration, industrial pharmacy, academia, and other pharmaceutical fields in our society at large. The Pharm.D. program is for the public. Japanese are lucky because the government led the revolution in pharmacy education. Treasure your learning environment and become a seven-star pharmacist (care-giver, decision-maker, communicator, leader, manager, life-long-learner, and teacher) to serve the public.

        Fe-Lin Lin Wu, MSCP, Ph.D., Associate Professor,
        Graduate Institute of Clinical Pharmacy,
        National Taiwan University, Taipei, Taiwan
        Chair, Pharmacy Education, Ministry of Education, Taiwan
        Member, Board of Pharmacy, the Examination Yuan, Taiwan

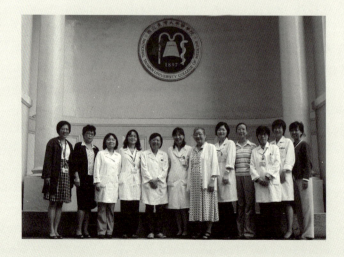

Chapter 14

Drugs Acting on the Eye

14・1 Reading

> 感覚器には視覚器，聴覚器，嗅覚器・味覚器，触覚器などがある．本章では，一般読者向けの英文医学書の中から，視覚器である眼の疾患に用いられる医薬品についての記述を読む．本文の随所で薬学・医学専門用語が一般英語に言い換えられている．今後英語での服薬指導に役立つ，患者さんにわかりやすい言葉を習得しよう．

Track 14

Many eye disorders are treated with eyedrops or ointments. Minor problems, such as irritation to the eyes caused by allergy, can often be relieved with over-the-counter remedies. Drugs that are used to treat infections and other serious conditions, such as uveitis or scleritis, in
5 which parts of the eye become inflamed, are available only by prescription.

irritation　炎症，刺激
remedy　OTC 薬，市販薬
uveitis　ぶどう膜炎
scleritis　強膜炎

What are the types?

The main types of drugs used to treat eye disorders are anti-infective drugs and anti-inflammatory drugs. Anti-infective drugs are commonly
10 used in the treatment of bacterial, viral, and, less commonly, fungal infections of the eye. Anti-inflammatory drugs are used to relieve the redness and swelling that may develop as a result of infection, allergic reactions, or autoimmune disorders (in which the immune system attacks the body's own tissues). Artificial tears are used to relieve dry eyes.
15 Mydriatics widen (dilate) the pupils and are mainly used to treat uveitis.

fungal　真菌の

autoimmune disorder
自己免疫疾患
dry eye　ドライアイ
mydriatic　散瞳薬
pupil　瞳孔

Anti-infective drugs

There are two main groups of drugs used to treat eye infections. Antibiotics, such as chloramphenicol, may be used to treat bacterial infections such as conjunctivitis and blepharitis. Antiviral drugs, such as acyclovir, are used to treat corneal ulcers that occur as a result of infection with the herpes virus.

Antibiotics are usually applied as eyedrops or ointment directly onto the site of infection in the eye. However, if a bacterial infection is severe, it may be necessary to take oral antibiotics as well as using eyedrops. Viral infections of the eye may be treated with both antiviral eyedrops and oral antiviral drugs.

When using antibiotic eyedrops or ointment, you may experience temporary stinging or itching. You may also notice a bitter taste as the eyedrops run down inside the tear ducts and into your nose and mouth.

Anti-inflammatory drugs

The drugs most commonly prescribed to treat the inflammation that accompanies many eye disorders are corticosteroids and antiallergy drugs.

Corticosteroids are applied as eyedrops or as ointment just inside the eyelids. If you are predisposed to develop chronic glaucoma, in which the pressure of fluid in the eye becomes abnormally high, the use of corticosteroids may slightly increase your risk of developing drug-induced glaucoma. Corticosteroids are available by prescription and must only be used under the supervision of your doctor.

Short-term inflammation caused by allergy is often treated with antihistamine or cromolyn sodium eyedrops. Some antiallergy eyedrops, such as those used to treat eye irritation associated with hay fever, are available over the counter. Antiallergy drugs may cause side effects such as blurry vision and headache.

Artificial tears

Eyedrops containing chemicals to relieve dry eyes are available for people who do not produce enough natural tear fluid. Artificial tears form a moist film on the cornea soothing and rehydrating the surface of the eyes. Artificial tear preparations are available over the counter and may be applied as often as necessary.

Mydriatics

These drugs are used to treat uveitis, an inflammatory condition affecting the iris (the colored part of the eye) and the muscles that control focusing. If the iris becomes inflamed, there is a danger that it may stick to the lens of the eye. Mydriatics shrink the inflamed iris by causing its muscles to contract, thereby dilating (widening) the pupil. Mydriatics may also be used to dilate the pupil during eye examinations and eye surgery.

Mydriatics are usually prescribed in the form of eyedrops or eye ointment. While using a mydriatic drug, you may find that bright lights cause discomfort and you may also have difficulty focusing. These drugs can cause contact dermatitis and may cause other side effects, including dry mouth, constipation, and difficulty urinating. Certain mydriatics, such as phenylephrine, can raise blood pressure and are therefore unsuitable for people with high blood pressure.

出 典："American College of Physicians Complete home medical guide" ed by D. R. Goldmann, 919〜921, Dorling Kindersley(2003). Copyright ©1999,2003 Dorling Kindersley Ltd. Penguin Books Ltd. の許可を得て転載.

14・2 Comprehension Questions

Based on the reading passage, circle T (true) or F (false) for each statement.

1. We may have to take medications orally for severe eye problems.　　　　(T , F)
2. Some anti-inflammatory eyedrops may run down into our nose and mouth leaving a bitter taste.　　　　(T , F)
3. Every patient may have an increased risk of developing drug-induced glaucoma after taking corticosteroids.　　　　(T , F)

14. Drugs Acting on the Eye

4. Artificial tear preparations activate tear production to protect the eyes.
   (T , F)
5. Medication to treat an inflamed iris may cause side effects involving the digestive or even urinary systems. (T , F)

14・3　Grammar

In numbers 1, 2, and 3, rewrite each underlined phrase into a clause. Number 4 is grammatically wrong. Explain what is wrong with it. Translate the underlined part in number 5 into Japanese.

Target ▶ Clause

1. The overall risk accumulation is combined with the tendency <u>for cellular repair mechanisms to be less effective</u> as a person grows older.
2. Many cancers have a high chance of cure <u>if detected early and treated adequately</u>.
3. Some of the most common cancer types, such as breast cancer, cervical cancer, oral cancer and colorectal cancer have higher cure rates <u>when detected early and treated</u> according to best practices.
4. <u>Although we believe that the lead content found in our recent lipstick analyses does not pose a safety concern</u>, we are evaluating whether there may be a need to recommend an upper limit for lead in lipstick in order to further protect the health and welfare of consumers.
5. <u>Who gets depression</u> varies considerably across the populations of the world.

14・4　Medical Vocabulary

▶ 病気の名称と略語 (1)

Match each of the following words with its abbreviation below and then translate the word into Japanese.

1. arteriosclerosis obliterans　(　)　_____
2. benign prostatic hyperplasia　(　)　_____
3. acute myocardial infarction　(　)　_____
4. Alzheimer's disease　(　)　_____
5. chronic kidney disease　(　)　_____
6. coronary artery disease　(　)　_____
7. chronic heart failure　(　)　_____
8. acute renal failure　(　)　_____

a. CAD　　　　　　　　　e. ASO
b. AD　　　　　　　　　　f. BPH
c. AMI　　　　　　　　　g. CHF
d. ARF　　　　　　　　　h. CKD

14・5 Writing
▶ **Providing information (1)**

市販薬の英文説明書をみてみましょう．薬の主成分と効果や注意事項などがどのような英語表現で使われているかを調べ，書き抜きましょう．

Hints !
The active ingredients are....
It is usually used to improve....
Do not take this....

Name of medicine (　　　　)

_____
_____
_____
_____
_____
_____

COLUMN

目の中に薬を入れるには？

　点眼薬を差したことがない方はいないのではないか．では，目に垂らした薬はどこに行くのか？　まず，点眼量は1滴で十分．結膜腔は約30 μLなので，たくさん点眼すると鼻筋から口へ．もったいないが危険な話でもある．角膜表面に達した薬は5層からなる透明の角膜を透過し，前房に達する．無事通過できた薬もここで房水の激流と合流し，線維柱帯からシュレム管を経て細静脈へ．ある種の点眼薬が喘息や腎障害に禁忌なのはこのためである．緑内障は房水排泄系や，房水産生系が作用点なので，点眼による薬物治療が効果的な疾患の一つとなる．最近は，分子標的薬などの高分子のドラッグデリバリーが注目されるなか，眼科では，iPS細胞の世界初の臨床応用で注目された加齢黄斑変性症の治療薬に，抗VEGF抗体を硝子体腔へ直接注入する投与法が適応されている．白眼に直接注射するのだから驚きである．眼はいろいろな意味で興味深い世界．直径4 cmの小宇宙．鬼太郎のオヤジ，侮れませんよ．

（小佐野博史）

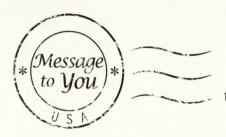

A Message From a Pharmacist Specializing in Cancer to the Future Pharmacists of Japan

Dear Pharmacy Students in Japan,

Hello, from sunny Southern California, USA! I am an alumna of Meiji Pharmaceutical University in Tokyo, Japan (Class of 2000) with a BS in Pharmacy. Upon completion of pharmacy school in Japan, I worked a few years in Japan and then came to the States. I received my Pharm.D. (Doctor of Pharmacy) from Western University of Health Sciences in December 2008. The school is located in Los Angeles, California. After graduating, I did a pharmacy practice residency or PGY1(Post-Graduate Year 1) at the University of California Irvine Medical Center in Irvine, California and my PGY2 Oncology Specialty Pharmacy Residency at Roswell Park Cancer Institute in Buffalo, NY. I have been a Board Certified Oncology Pharmacist (BCOP) since 2011. Currently, I hold a position as an oncology pharmacist at Kaiser Permanente San Diego Medical Center.

You may not believe me, but when I first came to the States, it took me almost forever to read just one page of a pharmacy textbook. I had to look up almost every single terminology. By the time I looked up all the words, I forgot what was all about. It was small step-by-step process probably slower than a turtle walking. Specializing in the area of oncology is very challenging but rewarding. Nowadays, one in two people develops some type of cancer. Thanks to screening technology, early detection and lots of antineoplastic agents in pipeline, we have more cancer patients surviving longer with cancer. Ensuring patient safety when providing antineoplastic agents is my number one priority among all others. And the patients are not only in hospital. They are everywhere because most patients try to maintain their daily lifestyle with their disease. We provide phone consultation for side effect management, oral antineoplastic agents etc. Having a conversation in a foreign language (which is English for me) is very hard, but I am used to it. When you're working, oncologist(s) just start talking to you even though you're doing something else, they may start talking to you from behind. A patient may be calling you on the phone. Nurses may have questions to pharmacists about chemotherapy or patient pre-medications etc. We need to pay attention to every single direction because you don't know when, where, or who questions are coming from. Some may require our response right away, some may require us to look and investigate articles. What I want every student pharmacist in Japan to do is to keep a positive attitude and grab any opportunity you may encounter. If your family member is taking a few medications, help them to make sure they understand the name of the medication, dosage, schedule and the reason they're taking it. Verify those medications' expiration dates. Try to check if they have any interactions (drug-drug, drug-food). If you find anything, bring them to the prescriber's attention or pharmacist's one who's working with the prescriber. Learning in English is challenging, but many pharmacy schools in other countries (including countries in Asia) teach almost everything in English nowadays at their pharmacy school. When you are able to communicate in English, you will open a door to broaden your horizons.

I hope my message to you enlightens your pharmacy career path.

Best regards,

Chieko Otomo, Pharm.D., BCOP
Kaiser Permanente San Diego Medical Center

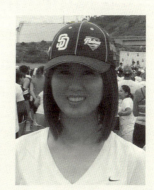

Chapter 15
Primary Isoniazid Prophylaxis Against Tuberculosis in HIV-Exposed Children

15・1 Reading

世界では，ヒト免疫不全ウイルス（HIV）に感染している子供の約9割がサハラ以南アフリカに集中している．この地域には結核が蔓延しており，HIVの流行がその状況を増悪させている．HIV感染のリスクがある乳児の結核感染および発症を予防するために，アフリカと米国の科学者たちが行った臨床試験の論文を読んでみよう．

exposed 曝露された

human immunodeficiency virus (HIV) ヒト免疫不全ウイルス

tuberculosis 結核

double-blind 二重盲検．被験者，研究実施者ともに介入（治療）群・対照（プラセボ）群の割り付けを知りえない状態

randomized 無作為化

placebo-controlled プラセボを対照とした

pre-exposure 曝露前

isoniazid イソニアジド（イソニコチン酸ヒドラジド；INH）〈結核の予防や治療の第一選択薬である有機化合物〉

prophylaxis against ～の予防

perinatal 周産期の（妊娠22週から生後満7日未満までの）

matching placebo 治療群と年齢，性，人種などいくつかの背景が同じになるように選びマッチさせたプラセボ群

Abstract

Background

The dual epidemic of human immunodeficiency virus (HIV) and tuberculosis is a major cause of sickness and death in sub-Saharan Africa. We conducted a double-blind, randomized, placebo-controlled trial of pre-exposure isoniazid prophylaxis against tuberculosis in HIV-infected children and uninfected children exposed to HIV during the perinatal period.

Methods

We randomly assigned 548 HIV-infected and 804 HIV-uninfected infants (91 to 120 days of age) to isoniazid (10 to 20 mg per kilogram of body weight per day) or a matching placebo for 96 weeks. All patients received bacille Calmette–Guerin (BCG) vaccination against tuberculosis within 30 days after birth. HIV-infected children had access to antiretroviral therapy. The primary outcome measures were tuberculosis disease and death in HIV-infected children and latent tuberculosis infection, tuberculosis disease, and death in HIV-uninfected children within 96 to 108 weeks after randomization.

Results

Antiretroviral therapy was initiated in 98.9% of HIV-infected children during the study. Among HIV-infected children, protocol-defined tuberculosis or death occurred in 52 children (19.0%) in the isoniazid group and 53 (19.3%) in the placebo group (P=0.93). Among HIV-uninfected children, there was no significant difference in the combined incidence of tuberculosis infection, tuberculosis disease, or death between the isoniazid group (39 children, 10%) and the placebo group (45 children, 11%; P=0.44). The rate of tuberculosis was 121 cases per 1000 child-years (95% confidence interval [CI], 95 to 153) among HIV-infected children as compared with 41 per 1000 child-years (95% CI, 31 to 52) among HIV-uninfected children. There were no significant differences in the clinical or severe laboratory toxic effects between the treatment groups.

Conclusions

Primary isoniazid prophylaxis did not improve tuberculosis-disease–free survival among HIV-infected children or tuberculosis-infection–free survival among HIV-uninfected children immunized with BCG vaccine. Despite access to antiretroviral therapy, the burden of tuberculosis remained high among HIV-infected children. (Funded by the National Institutes of Health and Secure the Future; ClinicalTrials.gov number, NCT00080119.)

Tuberculosis is highly endemic in sub-Saharan Africa, a situation aggravated by the ongoing epidemic of human immunodeficiency virus type 1 (HIV-1). The increased burden of tuberculosis among adults in areas with a high prevalence of HIV infection is also associated with high rates of transmission of *Mycobacterium tuberculosis* (MTB) to household members and other contacts. Therefore, it has been proposed that in areas such as South Africa, tuberculosis prevention strategies with isoniazid chemoprophylaxis, which so far have targeted only household contacts of adults with positive sputum smears for MTB acid-fast bacilli, be expanded to include other high-risk groups.

Among otherwise immunocompetent children, MTB infection in the first 2 years of life is associated with a 43% risk of the development of tuberculosis during the next 12 months. Also, the risk of culture-confirmed tuberculosis is increased by a factor of more than 20 among HIV-infected children under 2 years of age. Furthermore, postmortem studies have identified tuberculosis as a leading cause of death in HIV-infected children in Africa, accounting for 12 to 18% of deaths in these children. Isoniazid has shown effectiveness in preventing progression to tuberculosis disease in children who had known contact with persons with infectious tuberculosis, but its role in pre-exposure prophylaxis has not been evaluated in HIV-infected infants or uninfected children exposed to HIV during the perinatal period — both groups at increased risk for tuberculosis.

Our study evaluated the safety and efficacy of isoniazid versus a placebo for pre-exposure prophylaxis against tuberculosis in HIV-infected children and uninfected children exposed to HIV during the perinatal period, when treatment was started at 3 to 4 months of age and continued for 96 weeks.

15・2 Comprehension Questions

Answer the following questions in English.

1. Describe the risks to children's health in Africa.

2. What is the objective of this study?

3. What kind of study design was used in the trial?

4. Describe the details of the two study groups.

5. What was the conclusion of this study?

15・3 Grammar

Put the appropriate relative pronoun in each set of parentheses.

Target ▶ Relative Pronoun

1. Asthma is a major noncommunicable disease characterized by recurrent attacks of breathlessness and wheezing, (　　) vary in severity and frequency from person to person.

    noncommunicable 非伝染性の

2. One defining feature of cancer is the rapid creation of abnormal cells that grow beyond their usual boundaries, and (　　) can then invade adjoining parts of the body and spread to other organs.
3. The nature of the help or care has been further defined as 'beyond (　　) would be expected by virtue of family or social ties'.
4. While all of these products have been discontinued and are no longer available, there are a few remaining manufacturers (　　) have not taken the necessary administrative steps to voluntarily withdraw their applications.
5. According to one study of youth smokers between the ages of 13 and 18, 52% of smokers (　　) had heard of flavored cigarettes reported interest in trying them.

15・4 Medical Vocabulary

▶ 病気の名称と略語 (2)

Match each of the following words with its abbreviation below and then translate the word into Japanese.

1. disseminate intravascular coagulant　　(　)　_____

2. erectile dysfunction　　(　)　_____

3. irritable bowel syndrome ( ) _____
4. diabetes mellitus ( ) _____
5. fat embolism syndrome ( ) _____
6. gastroesophageal reflux disease ( ) _____
7. functional dyspepsia ( ) _____
8. chronic obstructive pulmonary disease ( ) _____

a. COPD   e. FD
b. DIC   f. FES
c. DM   g. GERD
d. ED   h. IBS

15・5 Writing
▶ **Providing information (2)**

生活する地域とある病気の発症率の関係は密接なものがあります．また，伝染病が特定の地域で発生することもあります．病気と地域との関係を表現する英文を作成してみましょう．情報源を明らかにすることを忘れないように．

Hints !
... is prevailing in the area of ..., according to the data reported by ....

_____
_____
_____
_____
_____

COLUMN

サブサハラアフリカ

サブサハラアフリカとは，サハラ砂漠から南に位置する48の国々を示す．貧困や紛争に加え，HIV/AIDSやそれに起因する結核などの感染症の蔓延がこの地域の国々の発展を阻んできた．

世界のHIV感染者3400万人の70％はこの地域に住み，子供の新規感染者33万人の90％以上はこの地域の子供たちである．特に若い女性のHIV陽性率は3.1％と男性をしのぎ，他の地域に比べてもきわめて高く深刻な状況にある（国連合同エイズ計画，2012年報告書）．

国連は，HIV母子感染予防のグローバルプランの中で，2015年までに子供の新規感染をなくすという世界目標を立てた．抗HIV薬の子供への予防投与などで，この地域の子供の新規感染者は3年間で24％減少し，効果は現れつつある．

一方，感染症の蔓延は無知によるところが多い．感染症に対する教育と啓発を行い，自ら感染経路を断ち，感染予防を行う意識や姿勢をこの地域の人たちに根付かせることが急務となる．

（塩田澄子）

Chapter 16
On Being a Scientist: Responsible Conduct in Research

16・1 Reading

> 科学の発見は共有されるべきだが，かの Isaac Newton でさえ自分の発見の優先権を守るために秘密にしがちであった．こうした状況を打破したのが 17 世紀後半に王立協会の事務総長を務めた Henry Oldenburg で，初の学術雑誌を発行し，"最初に発見した者"でなく"最初に発表した者"に発見の功を与えた．同時に研究者仲間による"査読"制度も導入した．研究者は他者の研究成果を自由に利用できるが，出典を明記することが必須である．

Science is not an individual experience. It is shared knowledge based on a common understanding of some aspect of the physical or social world. For that reason, the social conventions of science play an important role in establishing the reliability of scientific knowledge. If these conventions are disrupted, the quality of science can suffer.

Many of the social conventions that have proven so effective in science arose during the birth of modern science in the latter half of the seventeenth century. At that time, many scientists sought to keep their work secret so that others could not claim it as their own. Prominent figures of the time, including Isaac Newton, were loathe to convey news of their discoveries for fear that someone else would claim priority — a fear that was frequently realized.

The solution to the problem of making new discoveries public while assuring their author's credit was worked out by Henry Oldenburg, the

physical 自然（界）の
convention 取決め，慣例
reliability 信頼性，確実性
suffer 傷つく，損害を受ける

priority 優先（権），先取（権）
credit 功績
work out 達成する
Henry Oldenburg
〈1618〜1677. 英国で活躍したドイツ出身の科学ジャーナリスト，王立協会の事務総長〉

出典：National Academy of Sciences; National Academy of Engineering; Institute of Medicine, "On Being a Scientist: Responsible Conduct in Research", 2nd ed., National Academy Press (1995) より許可を得て転載. Copyright ©1995, National Academy of Sciences.

secretary of the Royal Society of London. He won over scientists by guaranteeing rapid publication in the society's *Philosophical Transactions* as well as the official support of the society if the author's priority was brought into question. Oldenburg also pioneered the practice of sending submitted manuscripts to experts who could judge their quality. Out of these innovations rose both the modern scientific journal and the practice of peer review.

The continued importance of publication in learned journals accounts for the convention that the first to publish a view or finding, not the first to discover it, tends to get most of the credit for the discovery. Once results are published, they can be freely used by other researchers to extend knowledge. But until the results become common knowledge, people who use them are obliged to recognize the discoverer through citations. In this way scientists are rewarded through peer recognition for making results public.

Before publication, different considerations apply. If someone else exploits unpublished material that is seen in a privileged grant application or manuscript, that person is essentially stealing intellectual property. In industry the commercial rights to scientific work belong more to the employer than the employee, but similar provisions apply: research results are privileged until they are published or otherwise publicly disseminated.

Many scientists are generous in discussing their preliminary theories or results with colleagues, and some even provide copies of raw data to others prior to public disclosure to facilitate related work. But scientists are not expected to make their data and thinking available to others at all times. During the initial stages of research, a scientist deserves a period of privacy in which data are not subject to disclosure. This privacy allows individuals to advance their work to the point at which they have confidence both in its accuracy and its meaning.

After publication, scientists expect that data and other research materials will be shared with qualified colleagues upon request. Indeed, a number of federal agencies, journals, and professional societies have established policies requiring the sharing of research materials. Sometimes these materials are too voluminous, unwieldy, or costly to share freely and quickly. But in those fields in which sharing is possible, a scientist who is unwilling to share research materials with qualified colleagues runs the risk of not being trusted or respected. In a profession where so much depends on interpersonal interactions, the professional isolation that can follow a loss of trust can damage a scientist's work.

Publication in a peer-reviewed journal remains the standard means of disseminating scientific results, but other methods of communication are subtly altering how scientists divulge and receive information. Posters, abstracts, lectures at professional gatherings, and proceedings volumes are being used more often to present preliminary results before full review. Preprints and computer networks are increasing the ease and speed of scientific communications.

16・2 Comprehension Questions

Based on the reading passage, circle T (true) or F (false) for each statement.

1. Priority means the fact or condition of being regarded as a precedent to others. (T , F)
2. Peer review is the evaluation of scientific, academic, or professional work by experts working in different fields. (T , F)
3. Publication in learned journals is important because the first to publish a new finding is likely to get most of the credit for its discovery. (T , F)
4. By the time research results become common knowledge, people who use them should not name the discoverer in citations. (T , F)
5. Wherever sharing is possible, scientists should share research materials with qualified colleagues. (T , F)

16・3 Grammar

Put the word(s) in the parentheses into the proper grammatical form.
Target ▶ Subjunctive

1. It is therefore imperative that governments worldwide (makes) policies and plans for the future provision and financing of long-term care.
2. While the Nutrition Facts label has been an important tool to help people make better food choices over the past 20 years, the only major change has been the requirement, effective in 2006, that trans fat (be) declared.
3. The WHO has recommended that countries (develop) antimicrobial surveillance programmes to integrate data from bacterial isolates originating from humans, food-producing animals, and retail meats.
4. We wish to acknowledge staff in all sites performing resistance surveillance; the aggregated results from this surveillance have formed the basis for the report, without which the report (will not be) possible.
5. The MedWatch reports led to stronger product warning labels, urging that the gel (be) covered after application to prevent its exposure to children.

Nutrition Facts label 栄養成分表

trans fat トランス脂肪

bacterial isolate 細菌分離株

resistance surveillance 細菌耐性の監視

MedWatch 医薬品の監視

16・4 Medical Vocabulary

▶ 病気の名称と略語 (3)

Match each of the following words with its abbreviation below and then translate the word into Japanese.

1. pervasive development disorders ( ) _____
2. toxic epidermal necrolysis ( ) _____
3. obstructive sleep apnea syndrome ( ) _____
4. peripheral arterial disease ( ) _____
5. rheumatoid arthritis ( ) _____
6. overactive bladder ( ) _____
7. urinary tract infection ( ) _____

a. OAB
b. OSAS
c. PAD
d. PDD
e. UTI
f. RA
g. TEN

16・5 Writing

▶ **Concluding a presentation**

プレゼンテーションは，最後に簡単なまとめをして終わります．その表現例を英訳してみましょう．

1. 結論として，私の実験は他の研究結果と合致しています．

   _____

   _____

   _____

2. この薬の有効性は，今後，さらなる検証が必要でしょう．

   _____

   _____

   _____

3. ご清聴ありがとうございました．

   _____

   _____

COLUMN

科学者の品格と誇り

"人は誰でも間違える"，あまりにも有名になったこの言葉は医療人のこころと行動を引き締める．学術研究は，真理を探究し得られる成果を社会に還元することも求められている．ヒトを対象とした研究では，ヘルシンキ宣言などに示される倫理規範を踏まえ，人間の尊厳と人権を尊重し実施される．科学研究では，膨大な時間と労力，社会の理解と協力，そして多額の研究費を費やすことによってデータが得られることも少なくない．それゆえ，データは，貴重であり，知の財産を構成する．知の財産は，記録，査読，出版され，知の継承物となる．その過程には，思いがけない発見の喜び，思うように進まないときのくやしさや苦しさなどが積み重なる．データのねつ造や論文盗用といった研究活動における間違いは，科学者の品格と誇りをも失わせてしまう．学術研究の世界にも間違うことが難しく，正しくすることがやさしい環境整備が必要になってきているのか．

（富岡佳久）

Pharmacists as Health Care Providers in the United States — Current Status

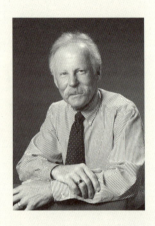

Health care costs are spiraling upward in countries around the world. Developing and defining a role for the pharmacist as a health care provider is a top priority. Pharmacists have been recognized historically for providing products in the form of prescriptions to patients. With the introduction of technology, there are increasing opportunities for pharmacists to provide advanced services to patients. In the United States, the pharmacy school curriculum includes advanced training in patient care and helps provide the basis for the provision of these services in many different situations. These include community pharmacies, ambulatory care clinics, and acute care institutions (hospitals). Working along with other health professionals, pharmacists now participate in the direct provision of care as well as providing prescriptions to patients. Examples of the type of care include: management of anticoagulation therapy, hypertension, hypercholesterolemia, diabetes, and other situations where there is a need for chronic management of drug therapy. In these types of practice areas, pharmacists are able to monitor, adjust, and select the most appropriate drug therapy for patients based upon their history, response to therapy, and laboratory assessment. Pharmacists in many states in the United States have worked along with governing organizations and other health professionals to change laws to allow pharmacists with appropriate training to provide these services.

Along with providing these types of activities comes the responsibility to demonstrate that in their role, the pharmacist does not add to the cost of health care. We must show that our provision of care is good and safe for the patient, and hopefully also decrease overall costs. For example, pharmacist-managed anticoagulation clinics have been shown to achieve better outcomes when compared to the usual standard of care. Patients managed by pharmacists maintain blood test results in the desired range more often, have fewer bleeding events, and this in turn helps reduce health care costs. In community pharmacies, pharmacists provide immunizations, health care screening, smoking cessation counseling, and soon provision of long-term management of certain chronic diseases. Providing access to health care is another positive outcome of the role that pharmacists can offer.

In order to expand the role for the pharmacist, universities must work along with professional organizations and governing organizations to promote this role. Individual pharmacists and student pharmacists must be willing to take on the responsibility to accept this responsibility.

        Steve Kayser
        Professor Emiritus
        School of Pharmacy, University of California, San Francisco

第 1 版 第 1 刷 2015 年 1 月 30 日 発行
第 2 刷 2015 年 2 月 5 日 発行

実 用 薬 学 英 語
(音声データダウンロードサービス付)

Ⓒ 2015

編　集　公益社団法人 日本薬学会
発行者　小 澤 美 奈 子
発　行　株式会社 東京化学同人
東京都文京区千石 3 丁目36-7 (〒112-0011)
電話 03-3946-5311 ・ FAX 03-3946-5316
URL: http://www.tkd-pbl.com/

印刷・製本　株式会社 木元省美堂

ISBN 978-4-8079-0865-3
Printed in Japan

無断転載および複製物 (コピー, 電子データなど) の配布, 配信を禁じます.
音声データのダウンロードは購入者本人に限ります.

実践的な薬学英会話集

薬学生・薬剤師のための
英会話ハンドブック
第2版

原 博・Eric M. Skier・渡辺朋子 著
新書判 2色刷 256ページ 本体2700円

音声データ
ダウンロード
サービス付

薬局や病院で薬剤師が，英語圏の患者に対応するときに役立つ実践的な英会話集．OTC薬の販売，受診勧奨，服薬指導，病棟での治療薬の説明など実際の場面に沿った会話例を豊富に収載．ネイティブスピーカーにより収録された全ダイアログの音声データダウンロードサービス付．

日本薬学会 編
プライマリー薬学シリーズ
全5巻6冊

B5判・2色刷（第1巻は1色）・各巻約150ページ

"スタンダード薬学シリーズ"の学習に必要な
薬学準備教育のための教科書シリーズ

① 薬学英語入門 CD付
本体価格 2800円＋税

編集担当：入江徹美・金子利雄・河野 円・Eric M. Skier
竹内典子・中村明弘・堀内正子

② 薬学の基礎としての 物理学
本体価格 2400円＋税

編集担当：小澤俊彦・鈴木 巌・須田晃治・山岡由美子

③ 薬学の基礎としての 化学

Ⅰ. 定量的取扱い
本体価格 2400円＋税

編集担当：小澤俊彦・鈴木 巌・須田晃治・山岡由美子

Ⅱ. 有機化学
本体価格 2400円＋税

編集担当：石﨑 幸・伊藤 喬・原 博

④ 薬学の基礎としての 生物学
本体価格 2400円＋税

編集担当：青木 隆・小宮山忠純・笹津備規

⑤ 薬学の基礎としての 数学・統計学
本体価格 2400円＋税

編集担当：小澤俊彦・鈴木 巌・須田晃治・山岡由美子

日本薬学会編

2006～2014年入学者用
スタンダード薬学シリーズ
（緑色のカバー）

編集委員：総監修　市川　厚・工藤一郎
赤池昭紀・入江徹美・笹津備規・須田晃治
永沼　章・長野哲雄・原　博

1 ヒューマニズム・薬学入門　　　本体価 4200円
2 物理系薬学
　　Ⅰ．物質の物理的性質　第2版　本体価 4400円
　　Ⅱ．化学物質の分析　第3版　　本体価 3600円
　　Ⅲ．生体分子・化学物質の構造決定　本体価 3400円
　　Ⅳ．演習編　　　　　　　　　　本体価 4000円
3 化学系薬学
　　Ⅰ．化学物質の性質と反応　第2版　本体価 4900円
　　Ⅱ．ターゲット分子の合成と生体分子・医薬品の化学
　　　　　　　　　　　　　　　　本体価 3600円
　　Ⅲ．自然が生み出す薬物　　　　本体価 4200円
　　Ⅳ．演習編　　　　　　　　　　本体価 3200円
4 生物系薬学
　　Ⅰ．生命体の成り立ち　　　　　本体価 4100円
　　Ⅱ．生命をミクロに理解する　第2版　本体価 5500円
　　Ⅲ．生体防御　　　　　　　　　本体価 3400円
　　Ⅳ．演習編　　　　　　　　　　本体価 4200円
5 健康と環境　第2版　　　　　　本体価 6100円
6 薬と疾病
　　ⅠA．薬の効くプロセス(1)薬理　第2版　本体価 4200円
　　ⅠB．薬の効くプロセス(2)薬剤　第2版　本体価 3200円
　　Ⅱ．薬物治療(1)　第2版　　　　本体価 5600円
　　Ⅲ．薬物治療(2)および薬物治療に役立つ情報　第2版
　　　　　　　　　　　　　　　　本体価 5100円
7 製剤化のサイエンス　第2版　　本体価 3200円
8 医薬品の開発と生産　　　　　　本体価 3400円
9 薬学と社会　第3版　　　　　　本体価 3600円
10 実務実習事前学習
　　　病院・薬局実習に行く前に　　本体価 5600円
11 病院・薬局実務実習
　　Ⅰ．病院・薬局に共通な薬剤師業務　本体価 5100円
　　Ⅱ．病院・薬局それぞれに固有な薬剤師業務
　　　　　　　　　　　　　　　　本体価 4800円

2015年4月以降入学者用
2013年改訂コアカリ対応
スタンダード薬学シリーズⅡ
（オレンジ色のカバー）

編集委員：総監修　市川　厚
赤池昭紀・伊藤　喬・入江徹美・太田　茂
奥　直人・鈴木　匡・中村明弘

1 薬学総論
　　＊Ⅰ．薬剤師としての基本事項
　　＊Ⅱ．薬学と社会
2 物理系薬学
　　＊Ⅰ．物質の物理的性質　　　　本体価 4900円
　　＊Ⅱ．化学物質の分析
　　　Ⅲ．機器分析・構造決定
3 化学系薬学
　　＊Ⅰ．化学物質の性質と反応　　本体価 5600円
　　＊Ⅱ．生体分子・医薬品の化学による理解
　　　Ⅲ．自然が生み出す薬物
4 生物系薬学
　　＊Ⅰ．生命現象の基礎　　　　　本体価 5200円
　　＊Ⅱ．人体の成り立ちと生体機能の調節
　　　Ⅲ．生体防御と微生物
5 衛生薬学＊
6 医療薬学
　　＊Ⅰ．薬の作用と体の変化および
　　　　　　薬理・病態・薬物治療(1)
　　　Ⅱ．薬理・病態・薬物治療(2)
　　　Ⅲ．薬理・病態・薬物治療(3)
　　　Ⅳ．薬理・病態・薬物治療(4)
　　　Ⅴ．薬物治療に役立つ情報
　　　Ⅵ．薬の生体内運命
　　　Ⅶ．製剤化のサイエンス
7 臨床薬学
　日本薬学会，日本薬剤師会，日本病院薬剤師会，
　日本医療薬学会共編．2～3分冊の予定．
8 薬学研究

＊2015年刊行予定

（2015年1月現在）